BREAKTHROUGH

CHRISTOPHER
SEAN STEWART

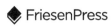 FriesenPress

Suite 300 - 990 Fort St
Victoria, BC, V8V 3K2
Canada

www.friesenpress.com

Copyright © 2021 by Christopher Sean Stewart
First Edition — 2021

All rights reserved.

ISBN
978-1-5255-6664-6 (Hardcover)
978-1-5255-6665-3 (Paperback)
978-1-5255-6666-0 (eBook)

1. BIOGRAPHY & AUTOBIOGRAPHY, PERSONAL MEMOIRS

Distributed to the trade by The Ingram Book Company

I'd like to take this moment to thank my family and friends for the support they gave me when I was diagnosed. I would not have made it without you. The countless rounds of chemo, the surgeries that gave me so much pain, and the radiation that burned me inside out. The aftermath was awful. I often thought: How would a brain damaged twenty-year-old ever be able to keep up? How would I ever make it? Every day was filled with uncertainty, fear, and rejection. You, my cheer squad, got me through it. Thank you.

BREAKTHROUGH

ON JULY THE 13TH, I ALMOST DIED.

But that's OK. It was an opportunity to learn more about people and life. A second chance to live, an opening to makeover the impossible, a foundation to make the impossible possible. Through this book, I hope to give you some insight into the things I've learned through my battle with cancer. I hope to give you faith that while life will never be perfect, it can become something that holds beauty and meaning.

After cancer, I lost three years of my life—three years that I should have been studying, working, drinking, and dating. Three years, gone. But I believed I could still do something great, despite my flaws. I spent many days grinding, looking for a way out, a breakthrough moment. Where I could prove to everyone else that

"I did it." The flaw in my thinking was that I assumed that everyone else's lives were so great, and even perfect. How wrong I was.

Everyone has their own struggles, their own pasts that haunt them, or that will. It just so happened that my struggle being cancer was in plain sight, while everyone else could hide their own struggles. But the only way to break through and become a better person is to accept who you are. Accept every single part of it. We've become so obsessed with other people's lives and standing up for the rights of others that we have forgotten to take care of ourselves first.

I want this book to give you faith in yourself. That you can get what you want out of your life, but you're going to have to accept all the downfalls that come along with it. There will be screw-ups and mistakes, but that's a part of life. With one missed door, a thousand others open up. So, keep setting that alarm, keep waking up because you owe it to yourself. And nobody's going to do it for you but you.

Use this book as a guide of inspiration when needed. You have all the success already built up within you. You just haven't found it yet. I invite you to take your time, take notes when needed, and discover parts of yourself you didn't even know that you had. There's a wall stopping you from believing in yourself. Blocking you from who you really are. It's time to break through that wall. It's time to be who you were always destined to be. That person is you.

SO FAR AWAY

ON JULY THE 13TH, I WAS SO FAR AWAY.

So far away from the dreams I wanted to chase. I almost died at 18 years old, with such little understanding of people or the world. I was passionate about people, good times, and unforgettable memories. But it only takes a moment for it all to be taken away. Love the people you have; love the places you see. It might not be ideal, but you're living the dream. There's pain, loss, and disappointment to be had. But there's always a light in the darkness, no matter how dark it is. On July the 13th, things got dark. But it's the one who steps back into the light when engulfed by the dark that survives to live another day. Live life, love life, every single day you can manage. Be grateful for what you have, for not everybody has it. Wake up and live with motivation, drive, and passion.

The following notes were written by my father, documenting the events that occurred when I had emergency brain surgery and was put into an induced coma. My father's notes are recorded in a separate font to make events easier to follow.

ENT Day - Wednesday, July 12, 2017

I woke up with optimism today. Christopher had been sick since October 2016. And things really started to progress May 6, 2017 when I took Christopher to Emerge to stop a nosebleed. Today was the day of Christopher's ENT appointment. Finally, he'd get the help he needed. It took way too long to get him into the ENT, but at least the day had arrived. We arrived at Dr. Anderson's office, just before Christopher's 9:45 a.m. appointment. Christopher was weak and had been throwing up. He was barely able to walk into Dr. Anderson's office. But he made it.

In five short minutes, Dr. Anderson determined that Christopher's situation was much more serious. He advised Christopher's symptoms were more severe than could be described by nasal polyps. He told, Christopher, Claire, and I that Christopher required urgent medical attention. He referred to Christopher's growth as a tumour and indicated he thought it could be one of two things: 1) Juvenile Nasopharyngeal Angiofibroma, or 2) Lymphoma. Dr. [1]Anderson called ahead to the University of Alberta hospital to let [2] them know we were on our way. Christopher needed a CT scan of the head and neck. He assured us this would be done the same day. By 10:40 a.m., we were at Emergency and had checked in. I was impressed.

Claire had a 1:00 p.m. assignment in Leduc and left around noon. Within minutes of Claire leaving, Christopher's condition began to worsen. Staff came to get Christopher's

---

1   Permission from father to use his journal entries. Love you Dad.

2   Checked by U of A Hospital Staff member. Permission granted via email.

CT scan. I helped him out of his chair—he took about six steps and collapsed. I caught him. I wasn't entirely shocked at this point; Christopher had been throwing up. He was weak and dehydrated. And had been sleeping. He was just put on an IV (intravenous tube), so surely, they would help. We transferred Christopher to a wheelchair and moved him into a bed in a plaster room. At this point, I began to notice behaviour anomalies. The doctor asked Christopher if he had headaches. He responded, "I don't know." I was floored—he had been complaining of headaches a lot. He also started making strange gestures with his hands. I pulled the ENT Resident aside and advised her that something wasn't right. She indicated it seemed that something neurological was going on. I stayed with Christopher and a very short time later, he appeared to have a seizure. I pulled the panic button—I needed help. Christopher needed help. I told the ENT Resident what happened, and they immediately pulled in an ER doctor. I briefed him on what happened, and he went into action. Christopher needed a CT scan immediately. But first they needed to stabilize him a bit.

I'm not sure of the time exactly, but around 2:00, we took Christopher in for his CT scan. I waited outside, for what seemed like an eternity. The doctor finally came out and told me I needed to come with him because we had a big problem. He told me that Christopher had a large tumour and that he needed to review his CT scan with me. He told me there were several scenarios, but all were bad. I was terrified. Actually, terrified doesn't begin to describe what I felt. As I was walking, Claire texted to advise she was back at the hospital. I asked the doctor to give me two minutes to get Claire. He showed us the CT scan which revealed Christopher's tumour was in his brain, sinuses and lymph glands. We were told that his situation was complicated and that they did not know how they were going to remove it. I broke down and the doctor's eyes filled with tears. The situation was serious, and we all knew it. Joint consult began between neurosurgery and ENT. We were both shattered.

Neuro ICU Day - Wednesday, July 12, 2017

Christopher was transferred to a trauma room in Emergency after his CT scan. We learned quickly that he would be transferred into the neurosurgical ICU as soon as a bed was ready. Until then, Christopher was monitored very closely. I'm not entirely sure what that entailed—I was in complete shock. Christopher's condition continued to worsen. His gesticulation increased. And his behaviour started to become aggressive. I explained this to the medical team as they had no way of knowing this wasn't Christopher at all. The doctor explained to me that, given the position of Christopher's tumour, it might be explainable. His emotions were likely suppressed. This also could explain why he earlier indicated he did not know if he had a headache.

Around 8:00 or 9:00 p.m., Christopher was transferred to the neurosurgery ICU. ICU is an intimidating place, but Christopher needed help. The next nine hours were very difficult. We were in ICU for a few reasons:

- Neuro and ENT needed to figure out how to remove Christopher's tumour.
- Christopher needed to be stabilized before going into surgery.

- The Doctors wanted to do an MRI before they operated.

The next eight hours were chaotic, emotional and challenging. I can't recall specific details of what happened throughout the night. I was terrified and overwhelmed. Neuro ICU is complicated. Lots of moving parts, all being monitored closely by staff. Christopher was never unattended throughout the night. And for much of the night, he had three or four staff keeping him stable. The key fight was keeping Christopher's brain swelling in line. Staff were constantly monitoring his pupil dilation and responsiveness. And adjusting his treatment when the results weren't what they needed to be.

At 10:20 p.m., Christopher was taken to the OR for a biopsy. More information was required regarding the type of tumour that Christopher had. Claire and I accompanied Christopher through the first set of doors in the OR and spent a couple of minutes with him while staff donned their gowns.

Sometime around 2:00 a.m., doctors advised us that they preferred that Christopher have an MRI before surgery. The earliest MRI appointment was 6:00 a.m. And from there they would proceed to surgery. But that they might not be able to wait. If Christopher's swelling increased, they would need to take action immediately. The other reason for waiting was there were more resources available to the team during regular hours than at night. As the ICU team fought to keep Christopher's brain swelling down, the surgical teams consulted on how to best remove Christopher's tumour. Given the complexity of his case, experts from Toronto, Montreal and perhaps other locations were consulted. Christopher had an operating room reserved. He was top priority for the U of A hospital that night. But time was not on our side. Christopher's brain pressure was not under control. The tumour was winning. At 3:45 a.m., doctors decided it was too risky to wait. Christopher had to go in for emergency surgery. Hospital staff started getting called in. At 5:35 a.m., Christopher was taken into the OR.

"When life threatens to take what you love away, that's when you discover who you really are and what you're truly capable of. That's when you become a true believer, an unstoppable force that refuses to give up." — Christopher Sean Stewart

Life threatened to take me away from my family and friends. It was going to take a lot more than multiple tumours to stop me. Because love was all the motivation I needed. Fuck the odds. Fuck cancer. It was time to do what many thought was impossible. Live.

SLEEPING SICKNESS

Christopher's Recovery - Day 1 - Thursday, July 13, 2017
I arrived back at the hospital around noon. I honestly don't remember much at this point. I slept for 30 minutes or so the night before and I received the most devastating news of my life. And had to share the news with Christopher's brothers. And now the long healing process begins.

Christopher was in a coma. There are three reasons for comas: 1) surgery, 2) medically induced, and 3) brain damage. The doctor advised he was likely in a coma from surgery alone, but his sedation would also put him into a medically induced coma. He did not think the brain damage was at play, but it's still too early to tell. Christopher was monitored closely for the hours that followed his surgery. I tried to sleep, without success. Christopher seemed to be doing well, but I hit a wall—I was completely overwhelmed. I remember very little of Thursday afternoon. Around 8:00 p.m., I left the hospital completely exhausted. I literally passed out at 10:00 p.m. and slept through until 4:00 a.m.

- Thursday, July 13, 2017

When Christopher was in the ER, I asked my parents to pick his brothers up. The boys knew Christopher had an appointment with the ENT on Wednesday. Initially, we told them that he was having his nose growth removed. Too many unknowns at this point. It was now twenty-four hours later, and the boys were worried. They needed answers. They deserved answers. Claire and I talked through the details and decided I would travel to my parents' house and tell the boys. Claire stayed with Christopher. I was to be gone for only for an hour. And was about to shatter their lives.

I arrived at my parents' house a short time later and sat the boys down to update them. I won't get into the details, but this was easily the most difficult thing I've ever had to do. I had no idea what I was doing. What should I tell them? How many details? Should I sugar-coat it? Why was this happening? I had no time to think this through. I had to get back to the hospital. I felt terrible. I was about to shatter their lives and run out the door, only to leave them with my parents. And my parents were only finding out for themselves. This was hardly fair. In the end I more or less gave them the same update as the doctor provided us. They deserved the truth—no matter how hard. I will never forget this moment. I want to forget, but I won't. And fifteen short minutes later, I left for the hospital.

BAD DREAMS

Christopher's Recovery - Day 2 - Friday, July 14, 2017

I woke up at 4:00 a.m., hoping everything was a bad dream. But that would be too good to be true. My night was over.

We went to the hospital for 7:00 a.m. We wanted to be there for morning rounds. We learned that Christopher's intracranial pressure (ICPs) became an issue at night. They had to hyperventilate Christopher around midnight and send him for a CT scan to assess swelling. No major issues with the CT scans and swelling was reduced through meds. Christopher was stable when we arrived at the hospital. Though stable, the news of Christopher's setback during the night hit me hard. The early part of the morning was difficult. I was overwhelmed.

Dr. Harris was responsible for Christopher's general care in the unit. His updates are fantastic. He helped me understand that you can't look at Christopher's current condition—because it's not good. Instead, you need to look at his progress in the last hour/hours per day. If his trend is positive, that's what you focus on. You don't think about what comes tomorrow, the day after, or next week. You'll drive yourself mad if you do. Dr. Harris always made sure we were aware of the little steps Christopher had ascended. And always emphasized the news was good overall. Dr. Harris gave me hope. And changed my perspective. For the first time my stress levels reduced—even if just a bit. But I also knew that this was temporary. I was on a roller coaster and emotions change quickly. But for the moment, I had peace. But I was also missing Christopher terribly. I wanted to tell him I loved him, and he was still in a coma. I sent him a text to let him know I loved him, and that he meant the world to me. I will be so happy when he can read it.

At 4:00 p.m., a social worker arrived, and I talked to her for nearly an hour. People asked if it helped. I'm not sure it did to be honest. But it felt good to unload. And I covered a lot of ground. In the end, I found out I was doing better than I thought. There's no rule book for these situations. But I learned I was navigating as well as could be expected to at this point. I've got a long way to go, but I've started to come to terms with how I'm going to deal with this. This doesn't mean it keeps getting better. There will be many hard days ahead. Claire and I are both fearful of the biopsy results. We need hope.

In the near term, hope will come from friends and family. On Friday, friends and colleagues started reaching out after learning of Christopher's condition. I was humbled by the response. In a world filled with negativity, lots of people wanted to help. I've never really needed help before. I was grateful, but also felt awkward about needing help to begin with. There are a lot of people praying for Christopher and for that I'm thankful.

REALITY

Christopher's Recovery - Day 3 - Saturday, July 15, 2017

Once again, I woke up at 4:00 a.m. wishing this were a bad dream. Only to be shattered by reality. Again, I felt helpless. I would give anything to talk to Christopher. Today I sent him an Instagram message. I'm sure he will think his dad is a fool. But this is what keeps me going for now.

I arrived at the hospital around 7:30 a.m. The good news was that Christopher had a good night. No setbacks. Yes! I was so proud of Christopher. And so grateful for the care he was receiving. But they had removed Christopher's head dressing and I was not prepared. What I saw bore no resemblance to Christopher. His head was shaved and bore an immense scar from ear to ear. My heart sank. No child should be in this situation. My Saturday morning was definitely much worse than my Friday afternoon.

Dr. Harris did his rounds in the later morning. And once again, he saved the day. He had advised that they started backing off Christopher's brain swell meds and sedatives. And despite that, his ICPs were holding. That was great news. He explained that ICPs rarely become an issue once this trend is established. But he did warn us it could take until Tuesday for Christopher to awaken from his coma. His update was uplifting and helped prepare us for the days ahead. But they were also clear that this would be a very long journey. I don't care—we are beating this.

Christopher's nurse David was excellent as well. I had unanswered questions regarding Christopher's incision and the tumour extraction process. David asked, "Are you sure you really want to know?" I told him I needed to know. And he graciously helped walk me through the process. Maybe I'm weird, but this helped me deal with the shock of Christopher's incision.

Even after the surgery, I had done to me, I still remember David. The ridiculous jokes that bounced back and forth between us. David always had the ability to make me smile in the grimmest of situations. I'll never forget the things he was able to do for us. Thank you, David.

These are the heroes that our society needs. The people who are willing to go above and beyond for another chance at life. They gave it their all when I was in a coma. Thank you for the support you gave my family. And thank you for those text messages, Dad. It made me feel so happy when I woke up to see them! I was alive! We would do it! We would breakthrough together. I don't know how I'll ever pay these people back for the courage and compassion they showed my family. It's nothing like I've ever seen before. You are all amazing people who deserve nothing but the best.

Christopher's Recovery - Day 4 - Saturday, July 16, 2017.
Another good night for Christopher. Two in a row! No ICP issues last night. Even better, the nurse advised that Christopher woke up at 6:00 a.m. He was fully awake. Because he's on a respirator, he was agitated and had to be sedated again. But this is all great news! I held Christopher's hand and talked to him. He opened his eyes several times.

At 8:45 a.m. Dr. Harris did his rounds. We learned that it took three staff members to hold Christopher down when he woke up. Fantastic news. This means he's very strong. The doctor said it's time to wake Christopher up. Unbelievably exciting. This is going to be a very big day!

9:35 a.m. Nurse just asked him to wiggle his toes. Nailed it! I asked him to squeeze Dads hand. Moved whole arm. Big, big day.

1:00 p.m. Christopher was taken off his respirator. Awesome! Around 1:30 p.m., Christopher said his first word. Water!

4:35 p.m. Christopher called me "Daddio."

A big improvement over an hour earlier. Asked if he knew my name. Mumbled a bunch and said "fuck." Kinda glad my name isn't fuck. Lol.

For the rest of the evening, Christopher was nauseous. And rather disoriented. Early on, it was challenging to understand what Christopher said. But after the 7:00 p.m. shift change, I could understand most of what he said.

Christopher asked when I arrived at the hospital and how long he's been here. And he told Claire he was scared. I decided to spend the night, so he had someone with him at all times.

Christopher's Recovery - Day 5 - Monday, July 17, 2017

The night was long. Christopher was scared and disoriented. I suppose much of this was normal, given his condition, but to me there was nothing normal about it. I'm scared for my son. He is different and I don't know if this is because of his meds or surgery. And, if the latter, if the effects are temporary.

Christopher didn't want to settle. I asked him to close his eyes and think happy thoughts. What's the happiest place on earth Christopher? "Right here with you dad." I welled up instantly. He told me repeatedly, "It's OK Dad, it's OK." He said, "Come here and I'll give you a hug." A very sick boy and still thinking of others. That's Christopher.

It's almost 6:00 a.m. and Christopher is still fairly unsettled. I hope this improves today. It was a long night. I'm worried for Christopher. And scared for us all. There are many things I don't understand about Christopher's condition. I only know what I see. And right now, that's probably not helpful.

Just met with Neuro Doctor. Christopher is confused for sure. But he said that's normal. Somewhat comforting. I also learned the attending ICU doctor changes each Monday. I will no longer have Dr. Harris to lean on. Crap. We are definitely on a different path. And the nurse confirmed he was up all night. Thank God she sent me to sleep for a couple of hours. I was physically and emotionally exhausted.

Christopher was agitated this morning. Didn't want to allow the nurse to draw blood. Had to calm him down. He has been great with me. Thankfully.

Dr. Clark replaced Dr. Harris on rounds. Pleased with Christopher's progress. Definitely behavioural issues and confusion but absolutely normal given his procedure. We discussed that I was getting questions from Christopher. Doctor doesn't think he's lucid enough to ask and told me he wouldn't remember our discussion anyway.

11:31 a.m. Christopher finally slept a bit. Likely no more than an hour but that's something. He said, "Dad, I'm tired of being sick." Breaks my heart.

PROGRESS

Much better night tonight. I arrived at the hospital around 8:00 p.m. the night before. Christopher was resting inter- mittently. Still in pain and nauseous, but not throwing up as much. From about 9:00 p.m. on, he mostly slept. He woke up many times, but I was able to get him sleeping quickly for the most part. Overall, the night was much better.

One of the neuro doctors popped by at 6:00 a.m. Pleased with Christopher's progress. He can start clear foods today (water, apple juice, Jell-O).

9:45 a.m. Started Physical Therapy.

11:15 a.m. Dr. Taylor came by. They are weaning Christopher off his brain tube. Will take a couple of days. As long as pressure remains in check, they will take tube out. At that point, they will get him up more and out of ICU. And do some other scans.

1:20 a.m. Just feeding Christopher Jell-O and cranberry juice. His first food.

Christopher's Recovery - Day 7 – Wednesday, July 19, 2017
I just missed the neuro rounds. Doctor said Christopher is better on every front. He's recovering from brain surgery very well. Had his catheter removed last night which he is thrilled about.

Christopher was happy to see me. He said, "I'm sorry I've been so emotional Dad. The meds make me that way." But more importantly, he said he was happy. Because I brought your wool socks? "No, I'm happy to be alive." I don't think I've ever been more relieved. I was scared he'd given up. He asked Claire this morning if he is going to live. Very tough questions. That no parent should have to answer.

Good chat with Dr. Taylor. Wants to avoid discussion with Christopher till we know what we are dealing with. Makes sense. Told him the emotional issues and that Christopher was on antidepressants before. He would review whether he needed to go on something in a bit. Dr. Taylor mentioned might be good to engage a psychiatrist in conjunction with breaking the news. He gets it. But also reinforced Christopher is doing great. Battle 1 is getting him out of ICU.

10:40 a.m. Nutritionist came. They are starting on an IV mix, carbs, etc., due to weakness. He's weak, but he can eat anything. We could now bring snacks from home. The more calories the better.

3:35 p.m. Physiotherapist returned. Christopher stood up, very briefly. But stood up.

Christopher was really throwing up this afternoon. And very confused. Nurse (David) confirmed what he was given (by another nurse) an opioid. Which the nurse confirms causes nausea. Told nurse (David) he did better on Tylenol/ codeine mix yesterday.

The neurosurgeon dropped by at 4:30 p.m. Said Christopher is doing great. Will be calling pathologist again. Wanted report by weekend. Will be doing full body scan shortly too. Want to make sure no cancer elsewhere. Sounded like Dr. Taylor will talk to us.

Christopher's behaviour changed quite suddenly. For most of the evening, he would not talk to his mother or me. He seemed angry. His jaw was clenched. He was withdrawn. Around 8-8:30 his mood improved dramatically. He started to smile. But when he watched TV, he seemed to look right through it. He was watching T.V. I asked what he was watching, and he said American Rejects. And went on to talk about the show at some length.

9:30 p.m. Just got a piece of toast down. Yeah, Christopher!!!

Christopher's Recovery - Day 8 - Thursday, July 20, 2017
One long and hard night so far. Just dozed off and Christopher decided he was going somewhere. Set off alarms all over the place. Settled. Then pee. Settled. Then vomit. Changed clothes and settled. And vomited.

But the nurse saw his behaviour as we do. Told me psychosis is potential side effect of his steroid. I told her I think you are onto something. She's talking to the doctor tomorrow. I thanked her. I'm all but certain she is right.

Another pee break. Then 3:45 a.m. blood work. No sleep for me tonight.

Christopher is suffering. I'm really afraid about his biopsy results. One week ago, I learned my baby has cancer. But he's had it for a while. This is the scariest fucking thing you could imagine. I can't begin to describe how this feels.

6:15 a.m. Just saw Dr. Very pleased with Christopher's progress. Increased threshold on ICP thing. Expects that it can be removed Saturday. At this point, we can take him out of the ICU. Christopher going for full body scan tomorrow. CT scan of brain on Saturday. Doesn't think drug causing psychosis as it normally causes persistent psychosis. Believes it's just delirium. Nurse told the doctor the night was terrible. Christopher will get something to help him sleep tonight.

Talked to Dr. Clark briefly around 7:00 a.m. Overheard Dr.

Alan ask if pathology report is in. Couldn't hear the details, but sounded like he said preliminary report is in. And results surprisingly positive. But wasn't clear this discussion was about Christopher. I asked the nurse if his prelim pathology report was back. She said she didn't know and even if she did, she wasn't qualified to comment.

Sometime around 10:30 a.m., the Unit Nurse came to see me. Claire wasn't here. Super nice lady. I learned that they weren't sure Christopher would wake up from surgery. I learned the staff were all worried sick for Christopher. And I learned that Christopher's tumour was the most responsive to radiation. But she said she didn't know how long he had. She ripped my heart from my chest. Claire arrived shortly thereafter, and I told her the news. We are devastated. Completely devastated. But united in our decision not to quit.

Christopher's Recovery - Day 9 - Friday, July 21, 2017
Arrived 7:00 a.m. Christopher had a great night. He was 100 percent Christopher this morning. "His night nurse Danielle, …" was exactly what Christopher needed. She talked to him about what happened. He Is aware he had brain surgery. He knows he had seizures. He knows he almost died. He feels very lucky to be alive. Said so. He's where we need him. He said it must have been scary for you. I'm so happy. Needed this.

Treatment will be a combination of radiation, chemo and more surgery. And will be aggressive. He's young and we're fighting this. Will know more next week.

Christopher's Recovery - Day 11 - Sunday, July 23, 2017

I arrived at the hospital at 7:35 a.m. Christopher was happy as a lark and eating breakfast. Big smile on his face.

Christopher mentioned his peripheral vision on his right side is forty-five degrees versus ninety on his left.

Christopher ate a lot today. Was great to see.

I remember sitting in the hospital, the faint scar that ran along my head, and realizing that my peripheral vision to my right side was gone. It was heartbreaking. But my parents' smiles were all I needed.

They moved me out of ICU. They told us they wished there were more cases like this. Most didn't make it. But most wasn't my family. I am happy to be alive, to be granted the second chance that not many receive. It hurts me to think that my life was almost over before it had even begun. Thank you to the team who fought for me at the hospital. You are all miracles. I wouldn't be walking if it weren't for all of you. My heart goes out to all of you.

A RARE CASE

Christopher's Recovery - Day 12 - Monday, July 24, 2017

Arrived at the hospital at 8 a.m. Christopher had a good night but threw up a little this morning—he said it was the pop he drank. He was up at 4:00 a.m. to use the washroom—he said it was really hard but managed to do it.

Christopher talked to doctor this morning. Christopher said he indicated multiple lymph nodes—not sure how many or where.

Christopher was very tired all morning. He had a couple

of naps and rebounded around 11:00 a.m.

Christopher's physician assistant, Lorrie, indicated Christopher's appointment at Cross Cancer is scheduled for Friday at 9:00 a.m. It will be a three-hour appointment. We need to come up with questions before meeting. And take notes as lots of ground will be covered. Lorrie advised Christopher's tumour is rare. As was the state of advancement when he was admitted.

POST SCRIPT

Moving forward would be tough. Many challenges lie ahead. Many of which would be devastating. But I can do this. We can do this. I'm a fighter, it's time to fight for my life. It's time to live.

THE POWER OF CHOICE

"New." A simple yet powerful word. "New." A word that had a major influence over me throughout my battle with cancer.

I had money saved away from previous work, but now—this was something new—I was not able to work. I had that choice taken away from me upon diagnosis. For the next three years, work would be out of the picture. Instead, there would be something new: chemo, radiation, and three surgeries would take work's place. I'd have a new kind of work—I was working for my life. And my chances were slim.

But! There is always more to life than just chance. My parents were told that I was not going to make it. But that never stopped my parents from believing in me. They stayed at the hospital for three straight days sleeping on chairs. They never left me. They were always there for me. It brings tears to my eyes, knowing that they went through that. No sleep, stressed out of their minds, not knowing if I would come out dead or alive. But that's the crazy thing about life. At any moment, it can all be over. One slip, one mistake, one cancerous cell that went berserk. It can happen to anybody.

"All it takes is one crack in the foundation. And that one crack becomes hundreds. Slowly but surely, the whole building comes tumbling down. But no matter how dark, how grim. There's always a choice to be made. To lay down and succumb to the darkness, or to push on to the light." — Christopher Sean Stewart

That day, we did the impossible. It wasn't my time to die. Life was barely within reach, but I held on. Why did I survive? My mom told me that I had always loved life. I believe I lived because I was unwilling to let go. I had so much love for the people in my life. Fuck, I wasn't done yet. I wasn't going anywhere, because my place is here. I belong here. My place is with my family. My mom, my dad, my grandparents, and my brothers. I could do it. I could beat it. Not by myself, but with my family. With my family, anything was possible.

To cancer, I have this to say to you, "How dare you try to take that away from millions of innocent families?"

So, while we were told my chances were slim. We believed in something greater than medical opinion or stats on a sheet. We believed in faith, family, and the power of choice. And the most powerful thing I could do was smile. Smile and show that the cancer wasn't going to define me. I wore that smile like armour. And with that armour. I was able to do incredible things.

And with a smile, I'm glad to let you know that so can YOU.

I've heard awful stories from people. I've met people who have struggled, and all I wanted to do was help make the pain go away. But I realized something. There are three types of people in this world. Those who stand by, those who drag you down, and those who lift you up to unreachable heights. I wanted to be the third person. I wanted to make people feel good about being themselves and feel proud of who they are. And from experience, I can assure you that it can be hard sometimes to feel proud of yourself. It was hard for me to be proud of myself. My mind would go to negative places, and with so much free time, I was able to create a narrative that turned me against myself. Each negative thought would lead to another. Tipping the next like a set of dominoes.

I like to call this the domino effect. The domino effect displays how one decision can impact the lives of many. A good example of this is how the stories of people overcoming adversity can inspire many others to face challenges in their own lives.

But facing challenges is often not easy. In fact, in my own experience, life's challenges can make you question your own capabilities, and perhaps even shatter your confidence and identity.

At twelve-years-old, I had an experience that shattered my identity and changed how I perceived myself. I was bullied. While I won't go into detail, I will say that the experience really dragged me down. The truth is, I felt so awful after it. I went home after it had happened and felt worthless. I felt so small, insignificant, and alone. Shit happens, and sometimes it can really suck.

While that one experience sucked, there were still plenty of good ones waiting to be found.

Prior to that experience, my mom found a Taekwondo

studio. The word is Korean, and I was told by my instructor that it means "The Weight of The Foot." After years of practising the art, I would describe it as primarily using kicks, technique, and flow. I was worried and nervous (as we all are when we try new things), but I decided to give it a go. I was so anxious, but little did I know that day would be the first day of a ten-year journey. I was given a white belt, and the class began. Yells of students danced off the white walls. The echoes of paddles and bags being hit rang throughout the studio. I loved every second of it.

We practiced kicking patterns called Poomsaes. Each belt level has its own unique one. They had to be remembered for testings. Tastings were held when students were ready to progress from one belt level to the next. For these tastings, students also had to break wood boards.

In order to get my yellow belt, I had to do a front snap kick. I remember that satisfying snap of wood as my foot went straight through the board, followed immediately by an applause.

I loved the belt system. Going from white to yellow stripe to yellow belt gave me a sense of progress. It also gave me a sense of achievement and pride. And at junior black belt, I won student of the year, the year after I was nominated and came third for the award.

Along with that, I participated in tournaments and won gold medal after gold medal. I eventually started teaching other kids. And I loved it. Encouraging kids to keep trying, to keep fighting. To see the joy in those kid's eyes. I look back, and I'm so glad I did it. I kept practicing and worked hard towards my black belt because I had a choice, and I made one. Seven years after becoming a white belt, I was given my black belt. A journey that would turn into a decade began with a single new decision.

New can also hurt. It's the silent assassin hiding in the dark, the ghost that haunts you from the shadows. It's always out there in some way, shape, or form. The problem? How are you supposed to fight an enemy when you don't always know what the enemy looks like? What does it sound like? Does the tension in the room change when it's present? The answer to that last question is yes. That's what makes "new" so scary. Because while new can bring happiness and joy into a room, it can also bring fear with it. And fear was a very prevalent part of my journey, and it's a huge part of many other's journeys as well. And in the past, fear may have led to closed minds.

Luckily, things have gotten better. Back then, society was more-close minded than today. Different religion? Convert or die. Different ethnicity? You're public enemy number one. Sexual consent? There wasn't even a concept like that hundreds of years ago. Now, look at us! We've swung the opposite direction! Which in many ways is incredible! There are numerous religions, many people are embracing different cultures, and from my own experience, many people are quite open to having positive discussions about their beliefs. We also have a variety of dating sites where you can filter out the things that you think are unwanted or unnecessary in your ideal relationship. There's a lot going on in our own worlds that we experience.

But at times, the world can feel like it's moving so fast. And It can be hard to keep up. We live in a world that is constantly changing and evolving. Where the only constant variable is the very change happening around us.

Ads flash up on TV and on our phones, tempting us, testing us, deceiving us. Black Friday, it can become a mob mentality. The mob starts with one person that posts the sale on social media. From there, it spreads like wildfire. And in a matter of hours, everyone can know what's going down. Being aware of the problems surrounding you is the first step. Without a proper diagnosis to the problem at hand, there is no chance at a cure.

Right now, as you read, there are people out there who are truly unhappy and unsatisfied with their lives. Let's say there's a man named Brad. Brad goes out drinking multiple times a week, and when asked if he had a good time. He always responds with a definite, "Yes!"

While Brad could be having a great time, it's important to note that when fun side activities become obsessive to the point of covering up our pain, it becomes a problem. Brad may need to ask himself, "Am I really happy?" "Or am I filling that empty hole in my heart with drunken nights because I am unwilling to admit that I am unhappy?" There are plenty of people who go to the bar and have a great time, but not everyone is going for the right reasons. Brad may not realize it, but he has a choice. And no matter how bad things get, you always have the ability to make a choice that will make your situation better or that will make your situation worse.

After my treatment, I went out to the bars with my buddies. Don't get me wrong, I had some fun nights, but there were many times I would come back home and feel awful. Seeing all the people my age at bars having a good time was a reminder of all the things I didn't have anymore. People I knew talked about school, work, and relationships. And I couldn't relate to any of it. I felt like a complete outcast. I kept trying to go out to the bar because I just wanted to feel like a normal kid again. The truth was, I just wanted to fit in. I wanted the life back that had been taken away from me. I looked sick from treatment, and sometimes other people feared talking to me because of the way I looked. And it hurt. It hurt to be treated poorly by others after my face had been disfigured from surgery. And at the time, it felt like I was robbed of everything and given nothing in return. But I was wrong. I was given wisdom and perspective and have been fortunate enough to meet some very wonderful people. And for that, I'm truly grateful. I did still feel unheard at times.

I just wanted someone to listen at a time when I felt so desperate and isolated.

But at some point, we all get desperate. It's unavoidable. At one point in your life, you will feel desperate. Kids playing arcade machines get desperate when they are just short of the prize that they have been working hours for. Guys get desperate when the girl they like is fading away. Girls get desperate when the guy they love has moved on. When you need to pass that test, and you are panicking for better study notes. Hell, we've all been there and if you haven't been there, trust me, you will. Desperation sucks, and when people get desperate, they can do some pretty stupid things. It doesn't matter who you are, your brain will go into fight or flight, and you'll do something really dumb.

But here's the bright side. You have a choice to acknowledge your good and bad habits. We all get desperate or feel it in some way, big or small. When we get desperate, we can panic and become highly irrational.

A man may rob a bank because he feels hopeless, like he has no other option. Stop giving yourself reasons for why you can't and start giving yourself reasons for why you can. I've got good news and bad news. You are your own biggest hero, but also your own worst enemy. How does it all change? With a choice.

Who is your hero? Who inspires you to be the best you? Many kids nowadays might say a hero with superpowers. Someone who looks badass does cool shit, and saves the world. As that kid grows up, he will have his own unique experiences that change his perspective of himself, others, and will redefine what a hero means to him.

Before cancer, I looked up to many professional athletes. Cancer changed my perspective of people completely. I still have respect for these athletes, but my heroes are the survivors I have met. The people who always found something to fight for when they had almost nothing left. And when I felt like I had nothing left, I looked for a motive.

With motive, there commonly is a source, a battery, if you will. A little spark that gets you excited. Gets the juices flowing and the heart hammering like a hummingbird's wings. A source of energy, a raging fire of compassion burning within every part of you.

That fuel source is inspiration. And throughout my treatment, I was inspired by not just the people fighting for their lives around me, but also inspired by the many stories

I could find online. That choice that I made (to dip into the inspiration around me) helped push me to keep fighting. But there is something out there that can stop us from reaching our full potential. It can stop us from making the right choices and from becoming the person we really want to be. And that thing that I'm talking about are the excuses we make.

EXCUSES

Ever try out for a team or perhaps even a club and not make it? After all the blood, sweat, and tears, the stars just did not seem to align. You feel angry, disappointed, and very confused. The days continue to go on, and echoes of the kids who did make it begin to bounce around the walls of the school. With that, so many things come to mind. We may feel like a loser, like our life has gone up in flames, and there is no coming back from it.

This is how many may feel when falling short. And it's so easy to look at this kid from the outside and say, "Ahhh, there's always next year, Jake." But it's totally different when you have lived through the air balls that everyone else saw. Jake may feel like a victim and that everyone is going to look at him as "King Air Ball." The sad part is, if Jake lets them look at him that way, they probably will continue to see him as the kid who never made the team. But that's not how his story has to end.

Take a deep breath in and close your eyes. Use that sense of failure, that sense of humiliation, and envision in your mind how you are going to break it. Do it. Envision yourself walking to the gym after school. Shooting hoops and playing with others. Watch and learn.

Sure kid, you missed out on this year. That does not mean you can't make it next year. What's stopping you from pursuing your goals is YOU. Sure, Jake got picked on by the captain of the team Damon. But is he the reason why Jake is not hustling? Is he really the reason Jakes not training every breathing moment he can? Nope. While Damon is an absolute jerk for making Jake feel that way, it's still Jakes responsibility to get back on the horse.

So, for heavens sake, stop pointing fingers saying, "The coach just doesn't see my potential." "These guys have more experience." "Maybe this isn't for me."

While others could have been blamed for my shortcomings. I sometimes had to suck it up and accept that the reason for my failure was my own excuses. Try your best to limit bad habits and start making ones that will give you fantastic results.

I, unfortunately fell to become worried about "the bigger picture." I began to panic when I realized how much stuff I needed to get done. There was so much on my plate. It was insane. All the surgery, all the chemo, radiation, and stress. How was any one person supposed to do this? How was I supposed to cope with this?

For many, what used to be an appetizer of chores, turns into a royal feast. Where now, not only do we have to take care of our own needs but the needs of others too. Amidst the precarious jungle of life are many obligations and duties. My number one duty should have always been making sure that I was doing my best to take care of myself after cancer. I became too worried about what other people were thinking when I should have been taking a breather and chilled out. Helping others is pointless if you haven't learned to first help yourself. What slowed me down was a boatload of excuses.

I've heard this from many other people, too—people from a more productive and grounded life. We all do it to a certain extent. We have those little moments where we can barely look at ourselves in the mirror. Where we wonder, what on earth am I doing? I sure did. I felt so confused and hurt after cancer. I was told that I was one out of only a couple thousand worldwide who had ever had this diagnosis. Talk about bad luck. I felt like I was being punished for a crime that I had never committed. And it hurt when I heard other people complaining about their petty little problems. I overheard a girl in a restaurant complaining about how one of her nails broke. She went on and on about it. Ranting to her friend, making it a big deal. And to her, I had to say, "Here's a full cup with a lid. Now, shut the full cup."

This girl, like many other people, has no clue what real struggle feels like. I sat there laughing and thinking to myself, *Wow, this girl is in for one huge awakening once the real problems come knocking at her door.*

I want you to know that it's normal to feel lost. To not have the slightest clue where you are and where you're going. It's normal to ask for guidance and to walk to dead end after dead end. I asked person after person for their advice. It led me to feeling hopeless at times when I still felt stuck. But a dead-end is still progress. And while it was not the victory I had imagined, it was one fewer road untravelled.

That, in itself, was a victory. I just couldn't see it at the time because I was so caught up in the worry of my life that had spiralled out of control.

Why did the appetizer of excuses become the feast? Because I let it. Life is very much out of our control. There are too many variables, and there is so much change that it's impossible to comprehend even a fraction of what's going on. The excuses I made were like quicksand. One excuse spiralled into two, then four, then sixteen. Until I had made so many excuses that I couldn't see a way out.

It starts small. Plan it out. I want you to physically write out what you're going to do and how you're going to do it. "But what if I don't know how I'm going to do it?" That's part of the fun. A plan is a general outline, a course, a roadmap that we envision. It is not at all a prediction of the future. You can't control your future. It's impossible. But you can influence it. Just like the future, an individual can influence how they perceive the excuses that come up in their head.

My mom suggested I come up with a road map. My road map consisted of simple tasks I could do to help me with my hand-eye coordination, improve my memory, and improve my physical strength.

I started doing occupational therapy to strengthen my hands that had been weakened by fifty percent from the chemo. My two therapists were Bev and Amy.[3] They are nothing short of incredible. Every time I saw them, I felt happy. All the excuses I felt I had, went away, and we went to work. Squeezing a strength ball between my index and

3 I've have gained permission (via email) from Bev and Amy, as well as their manager to talk about my experience at the Cross Cancer.

— 34 —

middle finger ten times. Then another ten squeezes in my palm. A whole hand squeeze, with which, I tried to squeeze the life out of that ball. Each individual exercise helped me, but the progress was so slow. So slow that I felt like I was going nowhere. But what kept me coming back were Bev and Amy. They let me play my music as I did the exercises. They were always open to jokes, good or bad. And let me tell you, were there ever some good ones. Over the time I spent with them, they did so much good for me. But the best thing that Bev and Amy ever did was that they made me feel like a normal human being. And after so many people had treated me differently because of cancer, it felt awesome to be seen as Chris. Not the cancer kid or the guy in high school who got cancer. All I wanted was to be Chris. And for that hour with Bev and Amy, that is exactly who I was.

I won't lie, the therapy was tough work. Especially the mental exercises where sentences were recited, and I had to remember and repeat specific details. It was mentally exhausting with a recovering brain. In my first surgery, I had part of my brain removed. In my second, my brain had been lifted out of my skull in order to create enough room to remove the nasal tumour and repair the base of my skull. I often felt frustrated knowing that I would have been better at these tasks before my diagnosis. I continued with it though. I kept trying. Again, and again.

My grandparents often would drive me to appointments. It took thirty minutes for them to drive from Sherwood Park all the way to Edmonton to pick me up. Without my grandparents, I would have been screwed. They drove me to and from, made me smile when I felt down and out, and never gave up on me. They didn't let my excuses get in my way. Their support was always in reach. I love you two. Thank you. I couldn't have done it without you.

It happens to all of us. There is nobody immune to excuses. The number of times I felt too lazy or hopeless to go to the therapies I needed, well, it's a lot. The number of times I made excuses for myself countless. It was my family that kept me going. That gave me the inspiration to see past the excuses I made for myself. When I thought I wasn't good enough due to my disabilities, it was my parents who gave me belief in myself. So yes, there is no immunity to excuses. I could either let my excuses hold me down, or I could carry that weight and put one foot in front of the other. I had to make the choice that I could do it. It's still hard, and there's still a struggle for me. But my job is to try the best that I can every day. I had to learn to accept that I would have to cope with the excuses my brain came up with. My problems weren't just going to disappear, and neither would the excuses that came along with them.

When I did let the excuses pile up, I felt useless. Like there was nothing I could do to better myself or my current predicament. I, at times, felt self-pity. The mind is a powerful thing. So powerful that we block ourselves from success with our own creative mental barriers.

Wall after wall we construct. Some of us have built more walls than others. Wall after wall, each with a line of excuses we've developed. Each wall needs to be faced. An individual must breakthrough that wall. Break the barriers they themselves, have developed over a period of weeks, months, or possibly even years. And over the course of my own journey,

I had built so many walls that blocked my way. But I couldn't give up because there was still hope. There was still a light at the end of the tunnel. I just had to get up and face the barriers blocking it. Every wall that I built could be torn down. And I kept going, and I kept trying, because more often than not, people are capable of much more than they could have ever imagined.

But now I've got a question for you. Who is your hero? I want you to imagine your hero. What do they look like? What are their strengths? What do they provide that can help other people? I want you to imagine this person doing amazing things. Not for fame or fortune, but for the good of others.

Now imagine having a figure like that in your life?! Perhaps you may already have somebody in mind. Whoever it is, this person can take control of a room in an instant. They achieve things that others would say were impossible. Now even though this person you have in your mind is incredible, it's important to remember that even they have flaws and have failed in order to get where they are today.

When it comes to failure, it can drown some of us.

So, how does one escape this foreboding sense of drowning? Step one, you must realize that you are not special when it comes to failure or negativity. Some people have it worse than others. But making yourself a victim and crying, "Why is it always me?" is not going to make your situation better. It is only going to make the feeling of drowning worse. Quitting is easy because anybody can quit. Your neighbour Kevin can quit, but Kevin is one hell of a trooper. In fact, the word quit shouldn't even be in your vocabulary.

Take a second and look around you. All the distractions. The clothing sales, all the advertisements being forced onto your brain, all the time and money slipping out of your fingertips because you are too busy making excuses. I had to stop making up all the reasons why I couldn't achieve my goals and start coming up with reasons for why I could, reasons why nothing would stop me.

Some of us sit around dreaming, planning, and praying for our moment to discover who we really are. To discover your own destiny. Fuck destiny. You are destiny. You are the author of your own story, and it's up to you whether that story sucks or is a home run.

There were long stretches of time when I got bored. I had nothing to do but recover after my body had been ripped apart. This time of boredom led to so many negative thoughts and excuses. Time after time, thoughts would come to my head. "You'll never make it back to school." "You're not smart enough after brain damage." "You can never live a normal life again." "You are not ordinary." My parents were with me to help challenge these thoughts. But the thoughts led to excuses. These excuses convinced me that I wasn't a likeable guy, and they convinced me I was not good enough. It was a vicious cycle. I kept looking for answers. I went to cancer support groups. I talked with others who had overcome adversity in their own lives. I read self-help books. They gave me wisdom and helped me think outside the box, think outside the excuses that kept me trapped.

And after doing all of that, I realized something about my own experience that is likely applicable to the lives of many others. That is, when you lose a sense of control in your own life, you want to get it back. After being diagnosed, I had lost that very sense of control in my own life. All my feelings of freedom were pretty much gone, as I was forced onto a different life path that I never saw coming. And while I had cancer, I desperately wanted to establish that sense of control in my life again. I hated feeling like my life wasn't in my own hands anymore, and it often led to feelings of confusion and frustration. So, in order to gain that feeling of control back, I did things to make me feel like I had a normal life again. I reached out to person after person, looking for someone, something, that would make me feel like a normal kid again. At the time, that's all I wanted. Was to feel normal and happy about being me. I chased people and relationships in the pursuit of happiness and a feeling of normalcy. But every time I tried, it never seemed to work out. It was hard.

The mistake I made was I was trying to force my life in a direction of normalcy because I was in denial about my current circumstances. In which I was unable to accept the way cancer treatment made me look and feel. As a result of not feeling good enough, I reached out to others in the hopes that it would make me feel normal and good enough again. But that obviously was a mistake. I was trying to earn the respect and approval of others before learning to like or respect myself. And when I had cancer, it was an easy trap to fall into because I found it extremely difficult to accept myself when I felt like my own body had betrayed me.

I reached out to others for months, and when I became aware of what I was doing, that's when I realized how much time and energy I was wasting on other people. I cared too much about what other people thought, and I didn't care enough about myself. Because when other people didn't call or text back during my diagnosis, I felt worthless.

How did I change? I filled in that boredom that led to excuses and wasted time and energy. I used an app on my phone to look at the amount of time I was wasting on apps. I had an average of three hours and fifty minutes on YouTube a day. Jesus. I mean, it was reasonable when I had cancer. In one way or another, I had to fill in the time. The problem was I had created a nearly four-hour daily YouTube habit which I no longer needed. As soon as I saw this, I decided that I needed to change.

I also reduced the amount of video games I played. I filled out a lot of that time in with going to the gym, writing this book, playing music, and instead of chasing happiness, I chased what I was passionate about. I mixed in moments of rest. There was no point in burning myself out. I took breaks watching T.V., catching up with friends and family, and cooking and cleaning. But once I was done my break, I got back to work. In all the work I do, I bring passion. With the writing came the dream of publishing. But now, instead of watching videos for four hours, it was time to change. It was time to take action and stop making so many damn excuses.

Why was I able to write this book and overcome the challenges life threw at me? Because I did not just dream. I got in the car, put my hands on the steering wheel, and drove. I was brave enough to get in and take command of my life, knowing full well that I could crash into a brick wall at any given moment. If you really want different results in your life, if you desperately want to change, you must be willing to own it all. Own the laughter, own the tears. Own the failures, wins, breakups, and mistakes. Own that shit, and you will be a force to be reckoned with. Every single day is an opportunity to make strides or excuses. But what will you do?

> "Success isn't money, status, or glory. Success is having the courage to fail, and the will to keep trying."
>
> — Christopher Sean Stewart

There are many excuses that come to mind.
"I'm too busy."
"I'm too tired."
"I'm too scared."
What is, what could be? Who could I become? That's exciting stuff right there. Excitement is a double-edged sword. Swimming with sharks would be one hell of an experience. Fascination and curiosity of these ancient creatures would race throughout your nervous system, fear would be provoked as well. Many exciting moments in our lives come at a cost. There is risk associated with it. That's what makes that moment exhilarating, breathtaking. A moment where two thoughts come to mind. I could die. But damn, this is cool! You still do it because it's awesome.

Jump in the water, swim with the sharks. Get down on one knee and tell her how much you love her. Will you feel scared and fearful? Absolutely, but that is to be expected. It's up to you to put your focus on the excitement that could come out of it. Not just the excitement, but the memories too. For the rest of your life, you will go around bragging, "That's right! I swam with the sharks!"

The excuses we make lead us down road B, when we were always meant to go down road A. Instead of going down a road less travelled, many follow a linear path that is "safer" and supposedly holds more promise for the future. It's less risky emotionally and financially. This is the fork in the road. The point where I looked down road A, where my dreams of publishing a book lay. But along with that dream came worries. What if nobody reads my book? What if critics think my ideas are stupid?

People have been judging each other since we lived in caves, and that's not changing any time soon. It was time for me to stop spending so much time thinking about all the things that were out of my control and would never change. Many of us will never even get to truly taste our dreams because we were too scared to throw the box of excuses out the window and pursue path A. Our true desires.

"I had to challenge the excuses and acknowledge that every journey comes with missed shots and missed opportunities. If you really do have a dream, you will do everything in your power to chase it. Having the courage to chase a dream is a dream in itself." — Christopher Sean Stewart

From an incredibly young age, we get good at coming up with nonsense. You were supposed to do your chores, but you faked not feeling well. I've done that countless times (sorry, mom). You were supposed to study, but you just couldn't get off your phone now, could you?

And as we transition to adulthood, the excuses we've developed come with us. You were going to go to the gym, but work suddenly became too busy. Your sister's birthday is in two days, and your answer is that you were "too stressed out." Really?! After all she has done for you, that's your answer?! We all get stressed. It sucks. Those "holy shit, my whole life just flashed before my eyes" moments. Hell, I've been there.

How about setting those stresses aside for her? Taking a couple of hours to get a meaningful gift that will put a smile on her face? Because once you do it, once you see that smile on her face. It will all hit you. "Damn, I'm so glad I took those two hours. Go me."

Not only do excuses get in the way of our dreams and self-development, they also can be crippling when it comes to our relationships.

When in a relationship with someone you care about, you should be a team. Teams have their ups and downs, like any other. And you're not making the playoffs every year. Some years, you won't even come close. There will be laughter and love. But anger and frustration may also be a part of the journey.

"I'm just going through something right now." Ever heard that one before? And of course, you ask, "What's the problem? How can I help?" And there's never an answer; it's always, "I don't know." They get angry when you're not able to understand why they feel the way they feel. It doesn't make any sense; it's extremely difficult to support the person you love when the best answer you get is, "I don't know." And that answer is totally acceptable. Because sometimes, we just don't know the root of the problem. Sometimes, it takes time, dedication, communication, and patience. But if you genuinely care about someone, you will do everything you can to make that time.

Balance in relationships is important as well. There are givers and takers. At a young age, we are naive. We think we know everything, but we don't. We think we're in love, but we've got so much more to learn about relationships. Failure is the key. Learning from your mistakes is key. Many successful people are the product of thousands of mistakes. The earlier you learn how to learn from your mistakes, the better. Because trust me, if you don't learn early, those mistakes will pop up later in your life. It's probably a good thing I'm taking care of that video problem now.

If you're in a relationship and the other person in it comes up with excuses on a regular basis. Try to work it out first. A lack of communication isn't going to strengthen the team dynamic you're trying to build. However, some people will not change. They just are who they are. Sometimes even though you love them, you have to move on. "But no, Chris, you're wrong, they can change!" No, they won't. Let them go. They will change for a week, then go back to the same things they were doing the week before. Your life is short, and you deserve better than that. So, start acting like it and stop letting excuses rule over you.

WHAT REALLY MATTERS

WHEN I FOUND OUT I HAD BEEN DIAGNOSED WITH CANCER, I FELT LIKE A TORTURED YOUNG SOUL. An innocent victim that did not deserve any of it. I found out from my nurse Danielle.

After waking up in the hospital, I felt confused and disoriented. My last memory had been at a high school graduation party with my best friends. I had planned to go to the University of Alberta and had gotten accepted. It finally felt like my life was going somewhere. The pieces of the puzzle were finally locking into place. The picture was blurry, but the prospect of it all was so damn exciting. I felt like I was on top of the world. Unfortunately, you can't feel like you're on top of the world forever.

Before cancer showed up on my doorstep like a vicious group of ruthless Girl Scouts. My life was stressful but pretty awesome. I had school, a job, a great family, and kickass friends. I was a young man (or a very large child) who loved doing fun things. My friends and I pulled off various stunts, and it was incredibly fun. There were moments where one of us would wipe out hard, and the rest of the group would hold their breaths, thinking, 'oh my god, did Jack just die?' Seconds later, when he would wheeze, "Holy crap," a synchronized chorus of laughter would break out from the rest of the group.

Love it or hate it, that is what made us, US. And that's what really matters.

There were also many nights of drinking and plain stupid fun. Everyone should have at least a little fun from time to time. Days where you just let go of all the stress weighing you down. A little bit of time to get some breathing room.

The conga lines, the music jams, and the tag that we played in the streets. Along with the neighbours who cheered us on from the sidelines of their homes. Oh, the memories of being seventeen and feeling fucking invincible.

Now, as dumb as that all sounds, this is what truly matters. Sure, you can chase your dreams and make a positive change somewhere in the world if that is an option. But there is more to life than chasing dreams. There's love to be engulfed by. Love that will irritate you from time to time, but there are people out there who will make you feel like you are more than a person. This person will laugh with you, drink with you, and will make you feel so appreciated. And you will do the same for them!

Throughout my diagnosis, I found myself being treated poorly by many people. My nose was crooked due to surgery, and it led to a lot of judgement from others, especially from some girls my own age. It was tough to deal with. Many people completely ignored me and pretended I wasn't there, and I felt so unworthy and alone as a result.

Who knows? Maybe these people had stuff going on in their own lives? Quite possibly, they were insecure, and maybe I was an outlet for all the rage because I was so vulnerable at the time? Regardless of all that, I still felt like a small and insignificant person, and if you have ever felt like this, you know how it feels. You can feel hopeless at times, a defeated, small, pathetic person. It sucks, but while you may be down, you are sure as hell got a lot of fight in you. You just haven't realized how much untapped potential you have within. You have a raging storm of untapped potential within you.

When I was younger, I had this very potential within me, but I didn't have a clue. I was not assertive enough. There were many moments when I should have stood up for myself, but I was too scared to. So, I took no action and remained feeling like a lesser person.

When you get trapped in a storm long enough, you forget what the sun feels like on your skin. You forget what it's like to feel like a king or a queen, and you become just another pawn in the game of life. That did not have to be me, and it doesn't have to be you either. You are a soldier, and it's time to stop being another piece in the game. It's time to move the game, inspire others, inspire yourself, and become the best you the world has ever seen. Even the alien life on other planets will hear about you. That is how epic YOU are. It doesn't matter if that person is named Dauna working at the supermarket or Kevin from accounting (Kevin is a total badass, by the way). Whoever that person is today is not the person that he or she could be tomorrow.

When I took this idea to heart, I realized that my today was the people who didn't see how awesome I was. And that my tomorrow could be so much more. I moved on. And you know what? I don't regret a damn thing. Today, I have great friends who respect me and laugh with me. These guys stood by me through all the fun in high school. They were there for all the high school drama, all the way to the classes where we talked about our next adventure.

But they were also there for me when I was bedridden from chemo—throwing up, too weak to get up. Through these experiences, I discovered it's not the people who are there for you when you are flying above the clouds. Nope, the most important people in your life are the ones who are there to catch you when you fall. Those are the people who love you, who are for you. After I had lost forty pounds from throwing up, I looked like a skeleton. My family and closest friends were scared, but they still knew who I was, and they still cared for me. They still saw me as Christopher.

That's what really matters, seeing people for who they really are. It can be hard to come by, but when you find it, it's magical.

There are so many more layers to love and laughter than you may think. Love and laughter are the purest, healthiest forms of medicine out there. Love and laughter will bind and heal the most traumatic wounds, both physical and emotional.

After Danielle told me I was in the hospital because I had cancer. It wasn't the fear that I remember over a year and a half later. It's the love. The memory of waking up and seeing my grandma holding my hand in hers. The weight of her hand was what mattered, and I'm so grateful for that weight.

Many more things come to mind. Seeing my grandpa and hearing his ridiculous jokes that made me laugh and lightened the tension when we were all overwhelmed by the thirteen IV bags I was on and the brain surgery that had just happened. My grandpa was and still is, damn funny. And fortunately enough, so is my grandma.

My mother and father are also incredible people. My mom always told me, "Christopher, we are going to get through this." She believed this with her heart. Her words dripped with nothing but the truth every time she said this, and let me tell you, having someone believe in you is something that you should never take for granted. Run to the hilltops and scream it. Share that belief and love with the world because it matters.

My dad is a trooper. He's the hardest working person I know. He has done so much for our family, and he puts those hours of work in because he loves us. Not only does he work hard, but he also pushes me to be a better person. Think about it this way. You've got thousands of awesome days left in your life to live. Each day is a gift, a miracle. Right now, you exist on a giant rock spinning around a ball of fire called the sun. I mean, come on. That's cool as fuck! Then, one day life just happened, and we eventually came to be. We fought wars, invented the cell phone, and for some reason, invented a way to sleep standing on the subway… Yep, we did that…Despite that, it's incredible that we are able to exist in such a weird, wacky, and wonderful world.

The point is, I would see my parents working hard, and it made me think *wow, I have an opportunity each and every day to make things happen.*

So, go out there and make things happen. Don't start crazy! Start small and gradually increase the risk associated with trying. That's all you have to do. Try! Start with something that is achievable.

Like, "I'm going to go for a walk today." Go for that walk,

play some music, and soak in the atmosphere. You're not going to live forever, so enjoy every second you can. Once you start to prioritize the things that are realistic you will slowly get better! Yes, that's right, you will start moving forward. Now don't get ahead of yourself. You won't be taking strides, not yet, at least. It starts with a leap of faith, and then you will start taking baby steps. That's exactly what I did, and it worked.

After my treatment, I felt powerless. Unable to walk or even sit up. I should have been moving into the prime of my life. But I was stuck in what felt like an eternal purgatory. So much work had been put in.

I studied hard for university, fought hard in kickboxing, and trained hard too. I had felt so fortunate that I was in the position that I had been in. One snap of the fingers and all of that disappeared, as if it was just a mirage in the desert, as if it was only ever just a facade and nothing more.

At times, it felt like I had been lied to. Nothing good could ever last because it always ended up fading away. I felt hopeless. But this was an opportunity to show other people that you can be bigger than the challenges life throws at you. All you have to do is believe and keep marching forward.

I wake up every day thinking about what and whom I'm grateful for. I'm grateful for a second chance, the people I have, and my computer for giving me the ability to write a story that I wanted to share. I'm greatful for my home and for music. I'm so grateful for the second chance at living my life that I want to make the most of.

Emotions are people's biggest strength but also our biggest weakness. How many times have we been angry, held a grudge, or even started an argument with someone we love? Eventually, looking back, we most likely thought *what were we even fighting over in the first place?* And it's OK! It's an unavoidable part of life. We all eat and breathe because we have to, to survive. But we also have to love and hate, fight and laugh, and do really stupid things.

Dogs wag their tails. Is there a scientific reason for why they do that? Most likely, but they do what they do. But are dogs hard on themselves for doing dog things? Nope. They eat their droppings, destroy, and eat almost anything they find and will pee in defiance. Dogs are just dogs. They do dog things. Do we try to change dogs into cats? Nope because a dog was born a dog, and dogs are simply better than cats in every single way. Yep, I probably lost a couple of readers there, but I gotta keep it real. Still here? Good.

Dogs take certain actions because they're just dogs. So, stop trying to be something you're not. Stop being a pretender. That's right, you don't have to be positive all the time. You're a human being capable of feeling it all. Don't let that build up because you are not perfect. You are human, so start acting like it. You will go through breakups; you'll play poker and will win some nights and lose others (trust me, I know). You will feel like a total loser one day and feel like Jesus the next. That is, at its core, what makes being a human being exhilarating yet frightening. Don't be afraid of the things that can happen. There are billions of people out there with their own unique problems. There are doctors, janitors, chiropractors, and so many other types of people out there. So just do you.

You know what else is often far from the truth? Our own expectations. Many people would like to have a fancy sports car or own a massive yacht. Unfortunately, not all of us will get those things. We all would like to wake up tomorrow and have our ideal life given to us on a platter. But things take time. Especially good things. It takes decades for trees to grow and develop, and to eventually tower over the rest of the forest. The same goes for people.

You start off a small seed that grows into a massive tree. But at one point, you were concealed underground, hidden away from the brutal weather that raged above you. There are so many new things around you that you don't quite understand. There is rain that pounds the forest floor, and at times, you feel like you're drowning. The wind is new. Wind throws you viciously left and right, forward and backward. You're not sure if you will make it, but you do.

As time goes on, you become smarter. Understanding of the world around you slowly starts to come together, and the world that once seemed like a mess is beginning to form pictures that actually kind of make sense. It won't be easy though.

First steps are exhausting. But in order to improve yourself, you can't simply jump from A to B. Marathon runners don't just wake up and start running 42K. That would be ridiculous, an insult to all the other people who had to sacrifice thousands of hours to get where they are today. You have to want it. You have to work for it like the other runners.

Let's call her Sasha. Sasha will start off maybe only running half a kilometre for the first four days. Day number five, however, she can run a full kilometre without stopping. Sasha keeps taking small steps and gradually increases how much she runs. One month later, she is now able to run five kilometres. That's incredible progress! Five times more than she was able to run initially. Sasha keeps gradually increasing the distance. Along with that comes the pain and agony of burning lungs, feet that feel like dead weight, and a dripping shower of sweat. But eventually, after one year, she is able to run her first marathon.

Why was she able to accomplish her goal? Because she was able to tackle it in a realistic way. Instead of going from A to B, Sasha realized that in between is XYZ-123. And because her mindset was in the right place, she was able to do it.

Post cancer, I was told that I might not be able to run again due to the side effects of intense chemotherapy treatment. I went through five rounds of chemo on two aggressive chemotherapy drugs. The first, Etoposide,[4] and the second, Cisplatin.[5] Both drugs were very powerful and caused a lot of discomfort, but both drugs played a major role in saving my life. If it weren't for these drugs, who knows where I'd be? But one thing's for sure. I wouldn't be here.

I'm so lucky to still be smiling, lifting weights, and playing music at twenty-one years old. I'm not done yet, folks. My gas tank is full, and I've got more amazing things to do.

The second drug, Cisplatin,[6] in my case, caused something called peripheral neuropathy. Neuropathy, more specifically in my case, peripheral neuropathy, is the result

4 "Etoposide," Cancer Treatment: A to Z List of Cancer Drugs, National Cancer Institute, last updated July 19, 2019, https://www.cancer.gov/about-cancer/treatment/drugs/etoposide.

5 "Cisplatin," Cancer Treatment: A to Z List of Cancer Drugs, National Cancer Institute, last modified October 7, 2020, https://www.cancer.gov/about-cancer/treatment/drugs/cisplatin.

6 "Cisplatin," National Cancer Institute.

of damage to the peripheral nerves.[7] Once the nerves in my arms and legs had been damaged, there were a variety of symptoms that I experienced.

Loss of sensation/touch due to damaged sensory nerves. Freezing in affected areas. Tingling and or numbness. Loss of coordination and balance. And a major decrease in strength and stamina of my body. Neuropathy hit me the hardest in my hands and feet, and unpredictable spurts of sweating were present as well. The crazy thing is those aren't even all of the side effects related to neuropathy. These are just the ones that I experienced.

I, fortunately, did not experience more, but I do still have a few of them. The important thing to note is while these side effects may limit my potential, they do not stop me. Fuck that. I'm going to live this life and own every moment I've got. And while you too may have limitations or excuses to make. It's up to you to keep moving onward. I wanted to continue to hustle, but my new limitations well…limited me.

The neuropathy made my hands and feet get cold. I didn't want to leave the house because I was so cold. Not to mention my immune system had been annihilated by the chemo, and my white blood cell count was literally zero. I'd gone through multiple blood transfusions and, damn, was that scary. All the things I had learned in school about what happens when you're given the wrong blood type—it's a scary thing, and I was petrified.

And, besides, all I wanted was to run again in the warm

---

7   "Nerve Problems (Peripheral Neuropathy) and Cancer Treatment," Side Effects of Cancer Treatment, National Cancer Institute, reviewed January 15, 2020, https://www.cancer.gov/about-cancer/treatment/side-effects/nerve-problems.

summer air. To be free of all the trauma. To be free of the stiffness in my hands and feet and the loss of coordination and balance. All because of neuropathy. And my hands were so weak. So, I could not write at that moment in time.

How was I supposed to live like this for the rest of my life? I felt useless. Like the used pair of shoes that nobody wanted to walk in. Each and every day, I felt sick. I was so frail, weak, and physically and emotionally broken. And all I wanted to do was run because that's what mattered to me. I wanted to get rid of the puke bucket, put my headphones on, and jog along the power lines with the sun shining down on me. I didn't care about having all that shit that other people wanted, like cool cars or expensive, overrated clothing. Nope, I just wanted to run. And while I could not run today, I kept my head up. I said, "maybe tomorrow." And when tomorrow came, and I still could not run, I refused to quit because I am not a quitter. But for now, I had to wait and heal. My time would come, though. It had to because nothing was going to stop me.

By making achievable goals, you will have a stream of many small wins. You will be drinking from the cup of success. Because you will get what you want. You went to the gym today! You started using sticky notes at work to become a more productive and organized person. You are effectively changing your life and focusing on legitimate, realistic goals that actually matter because they improve you!

I spent twenty-one days resting in the hospital with the people in my life who truly mattered. My family. There was so much that made sense now.

Prior to the diagnosis, it had all started with a couple of nosebleeds that always occurred on the left side. Never the right. Always the left. I would blow my nose a couple of times, the blood would stop, and I would go on my merry way. I just assumed that it was the dry winter cold. *Oh, another nosebleed? I've had one of those before, no biggie.* Oh, how wrong I was. I was so, so, very wrong. Despite the blood, I continued with high school, the laughter, and the fun in my last year at Scona.

For the most part, I enjoyed my last year in high school. The teachers were caring, compassionate, and damn, they were funny. I found the friends that mattered to me, and I had phenomenal teachers. There were great parts of high school. There were also tough times. And it's so easy to end up with the wrong people and end up on the wrong path.

Finding what really matters in an environment like high school is, for many people, impossible. In the effort to fit in, teens will do anything. Not everyone is going to come out better than they came in.

I had parted ways from one friend group, and it was almost Christmas. I didn't have a solid group of friends at that moment. Then, one day, I had a Social Studies class, and one of the guys mentioned that he was having a Christmas party and asked me if I was interested. I was hesitant. I was afraid that it would all be a pointless waste of time. But I gave it a go. That was one of the best decisions I had ever made. If it weren't for that night, I wouldn't have met all the people who mattered. Who stuck with me through my battle with cancer. All it takes is one night for your life to change for the better. That's what I learned that night.

This is the type of moment when you must catch yourself, slap yourself across the face, and wake up because what the hell are you thinking? Never turn something or someone down because you are scared of the outcome. Going back home and playing video games because it has a more predictable outcome? I was better than that. Scared and nervous I was, but I was brave for trying and drinking shitty tequila that night.

I met so many great people and made many friends that night. Every coin has two different sides, and so do the outcomes that are related to your choices. Hell, a different choice could have been made that night. I could have not showed up, not met all of those amazing people and instead played video games. The scary part? I would have never known the difference. Because sometimes all it takes is one tiny jump. One small moment where you internalize the fact that *what do I have to lose when there is so much more to gain?* It's often our own fault that we think this way. Our brain fears that one small jump because we've never taken that leap of faith before. We are scared because we don't know the outcome of the equation. That was something I had to learn. That more often than not, we have to just go for it and take a chance.

At eighteen years of age, I would be diagnosed with seven tumours. Many challenges would present themselves, but it was up to me to keep on fighting. I fought hard, and I lived every day to see the next because that is the man I wanted to be, and that is the man I would become.

So, run out there, soldier. Run out there screaming and make some moves. Feeling outgunned? Look for support. It won't be perfect. I stumbled and fell over and over again. What really mattered is I ran into the trenches with support. I fought with not just my head but also with my heart. And that is what really matters.

CREATING GOOD HABITS

WHERE DO YOU WANT TO BE FIVE YEARS FROM NOW? Twenty years? I want you to visualize it. Where are you? Who are you with?

Maybe you're on top of a mountain with your older sister smiling your asses off. You made it to the top! Maybe your heart is racing because you put skydiving on your bucket list. And the only thought running through your mind is, *why did I ever think this was a good idea? I'm going to piss my pants.* Maybe you're the best man at your best friend's wedding, and tears are dripping down your cheek. Yes, that's right; you are one sensitive man. Maybe you're at the lake with your buddies, all drunk, filled with laughter and memories. Or, maybe…just maybe…you just got lost while hiking, and you're crying out of panic…But don't you worry, your brother-in-law will find you and call you an idiot, followed by a big hug and a sarcastic joke.

Wherever you are, I want you to feel happy for that vision you're having. But slow down! Seriously, you're speeding in a school zone! Alright, pull over, you dreamer you, it's going to take time to get there.

Chemo at eighteen was not fun. It was hell. As I

mentioned earlier, my oncologist thought it ideal for hitting my body hard with chemo to give me the best chances. I agreed with her, and so the fun began. And when I say "fun," I hope you know I mean that in the most sarcastic way possible.

Chemo was received via a port that entered the superior vena cava. The insertion of the port was stressful. The surgeon doesn't knock you out for the procedure. Nope, that would simply be too easy. The patient stays awake, and while the insertion only takes about fifteen to twenty minutes, that doesn't take away from the fact that I was scared out of my damn mind.

Forty-five minutes before the procedure starts, the nurses recommend you take a pill that calms you down. You're supposed to take the pill before that time frame because, well, it takes time to kick in. In my case, they never told me, and so fifteen minutes before the procedure, I told the nurse, "I'm taking my medication." And that's when she told me I should have taken it earlier.

Going through this without it was extremely stressful. Luckily for me, I had another nurse talking to me while the procedure was being done. She was a wonderful lady, who was most likely in her sixties. She was actually very good at distracting me, but that didn't stop me from acknowledging that they were using a blade to cut into my chest and shoving a tube up there. But after twenty long minutes, I made it. An alien chord dangling from my chest. It felt bizarre, and if I'm honest, I did not want to move my arm at all.

Most people that receive chemo come for their treatment and go home. Mine was so toxic that I needed to stay put at the Cross Cancer facility for five days straight. That's where my new chord came into play. My chemo would go from the bag hanging on a pole. Flowing from the chord, the chemicals then travelled into my chest and into my body.

It all started with fatigue. Chemo made me really tired. I slept eight hours during the night and another five during the day. So, if you think your kid is lazy, they've got nothing on me. I was the king of sleep country.

Days were spent binge-watching Netflix, talking with family, friends, the nurses, and eating. For the most part, eating was actually pretty good. Keep in mind there are thousands of chemotherapies, and everyone's body is different. But overall, I did pretty damn good considering my situation. The nausea medications worked well, and for the most part, my stomach stayed under control. I occasionally gagged, but nothing came up. But when it did, my god, let me tell you, eating two McDoubles and fries did not go as planned for me.

Overall, I felt beyond exhausted, but I developed habits to keep my head in the game. I'd go for a walk around the ward with a pole I had named Paul. I smiled at the nurses as they passed. There were so many sick patients there. I knew cancer existed but seeing families and their loved ones struggling broke my heart. But I kept doing my walks. I plugged in earphones and blasted the Foo Fighters, Linkin Park, and Eminem. It gave me strength when I needed it most. And when I felt too weak to stand, my parents and grandparents were there to give me their strength. When I had all the happiness sucked out of me, my friends filled me with stories and laughter. I began to walk again. Back in my earphones would go, and back again, I would walk. Day after day, after day. It was slow. Really slow.

Comedy helped pass the time. Along with that, I also watched a variety of podcasts. What's so great about laughter is that it's an escape from whatever pain you're going through. For that hour-long special, there were moments where I completely forgot I was even in the hospital in the first place. Boy did it ever hurt when the special came to an end, and my eyes left the screen. The dream would end, and back I was to reality. But I kept up with my habits. I kept walking Paul the pole. I kept smiling when I could manage it, and eventually, the five days were up, and I could finally go home. It was the cherry on top, seeing home again. There was no place like home.

Surprisingly, I hadn't lost any more weight. Which was good. There weren't many positives, so I had to focus on what I still had. My family.

My mom brought me chicken soup, talked me through things. She built me up when I broke down. Find the people who build you up. You won't be able to connect all the dots along the way. But when you look back at your life and look at a particular moment. The dots will line up. "I get it now! It was so obvious!"

For dots to start connecting, you must start making better habits and get rid of bad ones. Stop comparing yourself to others. Stop thinking you wish you had Doug's life because you believe his life looks so much better. I judged myself so much when comparing my life to the lives of others.

One great habit I developed is I tell myself that I am an ordinary guy. Sure, cancer at eighteen is not typical, but at the end of the day, I'm a regular guy who happened to get cancer. And when I accepted that I was as normal as anyone else, that's when life became so much more enjoyable. Seeing myself as a victim only held me back. Cancer made me feel unordinary, and I felt like an outcast. But feelings aren't forever. I could still change my own sense of self-identity and perception.

Everybody is special in their own way. Some of us are great chefs. While another is a pilot, and because everyone is special, special isn't unique anymore. Special is ordinary.

I began to set realistic goals. I went for walks, worked out, and practised piano. And when I worked on those goals, more doors opened up. When you're able to achieve the simplest of goals and make things happen, you'll feel extraordinary for being ordinary. Make that a part of your daily routine. "I'm amazing. I'm incredibly ordinary." The sentence is structured to give you a dose of reality but reinforce that you're "awesome" and "incredible."

Purpose quite often can be taken the wrong way. Many people hear that word and start thinking about their life purposes. HUGE MISTAKE! We see others find what we perceive to be their own life purpose. We look at what our neighbour has, and it becomes a game of one-upping each other. And with social media, you have an unlimited amount of time to waste comparing yourself to others. Habit number one use your phone less.

How many times have you asked someone if they wanted to hang out, and they replied, "Sorry, I'm too busy." And maybe they are busy but perhaps not.

Another time-waster is our phone. It all starts with that

one picture or video, and once you enter, you can find yourself lost down the inescapable rabbit hole of online entertainment. The point is, those couple of seconds you pull out your phone adds up. It's an addiction, that dopamine hit you get when a text pops or the likes you get on social media.

In a guardian article, Parkin discusses Parker's idea of a dopamine hit (2013), "Whenever someone likes or comments on a post or photograph, he said, 'we... give you a little dopamine hit'. Facebook is an empire of empires, then, built upon a molecule."[8]

Now, you might be thinking, *no, that's not me!* Oh really? How much TV did you watch yesterday? How many text conversations are you in right now? And how many of those people are you texting because you would call them a friend? Or are they in the loop because it fuels that addiction you're starving to feed? More! More! You chase the high that you'll never reach. Your social status becomes linked to how many followers you have and how many likes you get. And eventually, your own feeling of self-worth may begin to stem from your level of social-media success.

Now, of course, this isn't everyone. But as time goes on, many become increasingly dependent on their phones. In many ways, our phones have become a third leg. We can't walk without it.

There are various ways in which I reduced screen time or turned useless screen time into valuable time.

---

8   Simon Parkin, "Has dopamine got us hooked on tech?", *The Guardian*, March 4, 2018, https://www.theguardian.com/technology/2018/mar/04/has-dopamine-got-us-hooked-on-tech-facebook-apps-addiction.

Number one. Focus on goals. Get a pad of paper. I want you to write out some things that you've wanted to try or do. Let's say Mike has always wanted to go kayaking in the nearby river. Mike should write that down and keep that note as a daily reminder on his desk. The next couple of months could be spent researching kayak equipment. Talking with people in sales to find affordable life jackets, helmets, paddles, and a kayak. There is so much adventuring to do. All you have to do is keep an open mind and walk out into the sandbox that is life. So, go do it. Write down what you want to do. Maybe it's simple, like trying out a new coffee shop. Perhaps it's adventurous, like exploring a new hiking trail outside the city. Whatever it is. Go do it. That new thing could become an amazing part of your life. You don't know until you try it. Make trying new things one of your habits.

I also turned wasted screen time into valuable screen time by using social media to share my experience with cancer. It allowed me to show others something very real. It was scary being me. I showed pictures of myself when I looked sick. I showed pictures of when I had better days. Because on social media, people post what they want you to see. Others want to give the impression that their life is fucking awesome. Guess what? I was okay with showing people that I've got imperfections. That I'm not strong all the time, that I'm not perfect.

My advice to you is to take out a notepad and write down who you are, the good and the bad. Be more open to being you. Make that a habit.

There are seven billion people and only one of you. You

are legendary, and there's no one like you. Own being you. Dive in headfirst. It could get messy and feel uncertain. But the beauty of life is finding yourself amongst the chaos.

We often tell ourselves *I'm not good enough! I don't know what the hell I'm doing!* Here's the beautiful thing. Nobody knows what the hell they are doing! There are many lost people waiting for their calling. Don't wait. Failure is the best teacher. I dare you to fail. I dare you to take a chance on yourself. Have faith in YOU. Go out there, screw up and learn from it, re-evaluate and come back stronger. The hardest part about fighting for myself wasn't the battle itself. The most difficult part was taking a chance on myself and telling myself that I could do this.

My high school leadership teacher Mr. Yonge had a very memorable drawing on his classroom door. It was a big white circle with an arrow pointing to the centre of the circle. At the end of the arrow, the words "Your comfort zone" were printed on the door. Above that big circle, another circle was painted, but it was much smaller. An arrow pointed to the small circle as well, with the words "where the magic happens" as the label.

We don't like pushing our comfort zones, but that's where our best moments happen. It takes courage to act. To push your own boundaries. Take a chance, go on that trip you've always wanted to take. Pick up a basketball and go to the court and learn. Ask that person out on a date. That act of courage could change your life. Do it for you. You got this. And there will be many moments when you feel like it's over. People have asked me, "Chris, how did you make it? How were you so brave?" The answer is simple. I never pretended to be anyone but me. I dropped the armour and faced cancer as myself, and taking challenges head-on is commendable.

So, I say this to you. You may feel like a loser now. You may be depressed or drinking too much. Don't settle. It's easy to listen to your emotions, but you must rise above your thoughts. Yeah, you don't feel like going to the gym? That's your thoughts talking, don't let your thoughts take control. Your negative thoughts do the talking, but you do the walking. So, start living the life you want to live. Walk that walk. Get up, stop feeling sorry for yourself and go to the gym.

I felt sorry for myself for a while. I had to heal, but continuing to sit around and do nothing wasn't going to lead me anywhere, and it won't for you either. Feeling self-pity is a bad habit. Get up on your feet. Everybody wants to sleep in, but it's not always about where you are. It's about where you want to be.

I wanted to run when I was told I might not be able to run again. I decided that I wasn't just going to run, I was going to fly. I showed up six foot two, 130 pounds, skinny as a rail. I was surrounded by people that were in great shape. It made me feel very self-conscious at times. Cancer broke my body and shattered my mind, but I was never going to let cancer break my spirit.

I felt so weak, but I was bigger than my feelings. I had a dream. I was going to fight and would not quit. I walked to the gym and showed up day after day. I was sore and tired, but I had a vision, and I was going to go where no other person had gone before. I took a picture of my body every day. I felt like quitting, but I refused. I pumped the weights and started walking on the treadmill. I walked the powerlines. I kept on marching forward. I was hungry for success, and I kept hunting. Two weeks went by, and I was still going. Then three weeks. Then two months. There was constant mental struggle and physical pain, but I am a man of my word. I told myself I was going to do this.

The noise inside my head would get loud. Shouting, telling me I could not do this. But I didn't give up on myself. I sucked it up because pain and struggle are a part of the process. There was no participation medal. The only thing in sight was the gold medal waiting at the finish line. The pain in my muscles got worse, but I chose to get out of bed and put on my running shoes. My balance (that the neuropathy had affected) began to get better. My strength increased. My stamina got better. I began to inspire myself. I felt proud.

Most people give up on going to the gym. If I can do it with my circumstances, so can you. There were ups and downs. I took pictures of my progress, and after three months of hard work, I had put on fifteen pounds of weight and a good amount of muscle. I posted a video on social media of my progress. It inspired people. In order to make your mark, you must develop good habits and eliminate the chains holding you back.

Be the author of your own story, write the next chapter of your life, wake up and develop yourself. Cut down the screen time and ask yourself who you want to be. Fight with the heart of a champion and rise to the occasion. There will be sacrifices that will have to be made. But if you want something bad enough, you will make those sacrifices. I did. And today, I still carry with me the habits that I've worked on.

Oh, it's freezing outside, and there's a blizzard? I walk. I feel lazy and unmotivated? I walk.

Some have gotten so creative at coming up with nonsense that they've become paralyzed in the process. Get creative with making habits. Open up your mind. Give more things a try. Don't jump to the conclusion that something sucks. If it does, ask yourself how you think it could be made better?

I was hurt by a lot of people throughout my healing. After going through hell, I just wanted to feel loved and appreciated. The number of people that saw me in a bar and shook hands with me and told me they had a lot of respect for me was astounding. And I did appreciate their compliments. They often would say we should catch up. And it gave me hope. But nothing ever happened. I would invite them out, but they would never invite me in return. I even had a couple of people ignore me.

Now, of course, this happens to everybody. But after talking with other cancer survivors, I soon realized that people just don't know how to treat cancer survivors. They forget that we are still normal people. It was hard to deal with.

On several occasions, I ran into an old acquaintance. I would feel excited to see them and waved. But to my surprise, sometimes they would turn their back on me, walking away as fast as they could. There were lots of people I thought who I expected to support me. Lots of people I thought could be a small part of my life. I was so wrong. I had some people turn their backs on me. And there were parts of me that understood. My situation was scary, and while I couldn't run away from cancer, but they could.

It's frustrating hearing people complain about their problems to me. I had someone complain to me about how hard their life was with school. I would have killed to have your problems. This person was likely to have a degree in five years, and I (at the time) was a loaded barrel of stage four cancer. Make a habit of complaining less and providing more. It will make you a better mother, father, brother, sister. Hell, it will make you a better person. Because while you complain about how hard school is, there is a kid out there starving who would be grateful to have an ounce of what you have.

There are countless stories of kids starving in third-world countries. Kids who go for days without eating. Kids who were convicted of nothing but being born in the wrong place at the wrong time. You, on the other hand, probably don't have it this bad. Sure, you got dumped last week. You got fired. But at least you were offered an opportunity to make something of yourself. These kids never had the blessing to make good habits. Your life starts now.

THE POWER OF STORY

WE'VE ALL FALLEN. Gotten bruises. Cuts. It happens no matter how strong we may think we are. As kids, we are unaware of how crazy the world can be. We don't understand that if we were to jump into a river, we could drown. Kids just see the river and want to go swimming. They don't associate any risks with their action because, to them, the world is a perfect place. A world filled with stories of fairy tales. To kids, heroes and villains are just "made up." They don't have the knowledge that heroes and villains exist because kids lack experience. They lack the many lessons that life will teach them if they're willing to look back and connect the dots.

In Northern Australia, the Patterson's had just become the owners of a beautiful house, and they were making their adjustments to the new place.

The parents were a lovely couple of thirty-nine and forty-one. Kelly and Nate had two beautiful kids who they cherished so-so very much. The oldest was eleven, who they had named Bella. And the youngest nine, who they called Mel.

The Patterson's had finally moved out to their new home. It was so peaceful, so quiet, and so perfect. It truly did feel like the right home for the family. The Patterson's even had a pond in their backyard. And ever since the family had moved in, Bella had not stopped talking about how excited she was to jump right in.

The sun's beautiful beams bounced off the pond's surface during the day, and it shone like white-silver glass during the nights.

In a place as hot as Australia, it was convenient to have water to cool you off. And for Bella, there was nothing more satisfying than jumping into cool water when the air around her felt like flame.

And after a couple of days, she finally did get the chance that she had been waiting for. As Bella sunk deeper into the icy depths, her body became weightless. And just for a moment, she slowly began to drift, and her mind went blank and still just like the water. With her breath held, Bella moved her arms forward and then backward as she continued to descend into the darkness down below. As her arms swayed, she adjusted to the heavy weight of the water that floated above her. Then her feet contacted the sand that lay below her. It felt soft as each grain slipped between Bella's toes. Then, there was a moment of peace and silence as the water became still. Then Bella kicked off from the bottom as she rushed back to the surface. Back to the people she loved.

The surface broke, and air rushed back into Bella's lungs. Her face felt cold but refreshed. Noise funneled back into Bella's ears. But each word sounded different as they bounce off the shimmering glass around her. Her eyes snapped back into focus, and Bella looked at her family standing on the porch, smiling with the brightest of faces. Her mother, with her bright blue eyes and beautiful wavy brown hair. Her father's neatly trimmed, sleek blonde hair. And her little sister Mel. Oh, sweet Mel. Her dirty blonde hair and her excited, stupid smile plastered on her face. It was all a perfect picture. Everything about it.

The house was a light pink with a light tiled rooftop. It wasn't big, but it was everything the Patterson's wanted it to be. And was exactly what Bella had imagined when her parents had described it to her all those months ago.

She loved it when Mel would ask her to play. When they would run with one another, their parents laughing together as they followed.

Bella smiled at her family waiting at the shore. But then she was sucked under the glass. She was spinning violently left and right, up and down. Water rushed in and the claw that had dug so deep into her leg dug even deeper. Then the world was gone, and she was nothing but a blank page. The beast had devoured her.

Stories are powerful. Not just the stories we read. But the stories that we tell ourselves. We tell ourselves various things every single day. Such as "I am confident." Or "I am attractive."

But the stories we tell ourselves aren't always positive. We sometimes subscribe to a different narrative. One that tells us that "we aren't worth it." Or that "we will fail."

Either way, the narrative that we develop in our heads profoundly affects not only our relationship with others but, more importantly, impacts the most critical relationship in our lives. The relationship that we have with ourselves. And when we don't have a good relationship with ourselves, there can be consequences. We may lack self-respect and not treat our bodies and mind right. Some might become more vulnerable to peer pressure as they don't have the self-respect to stand up for themselves.

But let's get back to the story I told. What made it so disturbing? It was the details. It made the experience feel real. For two minutes, you felt so immersed that you became that girl. It was almost as if you could feel the water as she jumped in, the sand hitting her feet, and the teeth sinking in. Anybody could have just told you, "A girl got eaten by a saltwater crocodile." Sure, it's scary, but it carries no emotional weight because there's no build-up leading up to the most significant moment.

By being specific about a scenario, you can pull people's emotions in ways you could not imagine. You can make people laugh their asses off and make them sympathize with you in ways they thought was impossible. And by making the impossible possible, you can touch people's hearts and warm their mind, body, and soul.

We all have dreams and inspirations. Sadly, some of us will never even try to pursue them. I want you to write down every day how you're going to take action on that dream because you deserve it. Every one of us deserves something to be passionate about. And I think you're wonderful, and you have a long life ahead of you and have a story to fill. Go take a painting class, try out volunteering. Take a little time to invest in you. Your story that you write for yourself doesn't have to be spectacular or outstanding. Love to live in the moment. Go out to the dog park, chat with someone new. Appreciate the food you have to eat on your table.

Every little thing counts when it comes to you and your story. Live in that moment.

As human beings, it's incredible that we are capable of feeling so many things. I hated feeling stressed out and scared after cancer. I tried to block out those feelings. But that stress, that fear, was a part of me. It's a part of you too. And I think you're capable of more than you know, and I don't want you to change as a person. I want you to change your habits, focus, and prioritize what you value because it will all lead to a better story that makes you. You.

As kids, we start off with big dreams, and as we grow older, our dreams get smaller as we learn about all the things that are out there that can emotionally crush us. I'm here to say fuck your fears, own them. I've been disappointed, pushed, shoved, scared, lied to, cheated, abandoned. But this happens to all of us. But I'm still here. I'm stronger, more resilient, and a better man. I'm going to keep on moving forward from one achievement to the next. At this point, it's ingrained in me.

How did I get there, you ask? I stopped dreaming dreams and started acting on them. If I wanted to write, I wrote. When I had questions, I sought for answers. I stopped fleeing and started believing in myself. I started a journey to discover who I was and who I wanted to become.

So, when someone asks you, "What's your story?" Do not limit that to, "I'm an accountant." One of our biggest flaws is that we grow up with the idea of having a "dream job" and that we have to settle. People's minds are complex. Our minds are constantly processing data and changing their wiring, upgrading, and downgrading. You're going to change. And while your hardware may be running the hard drive for an accountant for thirty years. Maybe the hardware changes and the computer begins downloading information about becoming a lawyer? But there's more! When someone asks Bill what he does. Bill will most likely respond with an occupation. "Oh! I'm a teacher!" It's such a waste to limit yourself to one word when you're so much more than that. "So, Bill, what do you do?"

"How much time do you got? There's a lot. I'm a loving husband, a father to three exceptional children, and a sports fan at heart. I also am a best friend to the most incredible guy out there. I'm a poker player who plays for bragging rights and no cash. I'm a jokester at heart, sometimes an absolute idiot. I'm the guy whose dance moves are unstoppable, an unstoppable force when it comes to love and laughter. My name is Bill, and I love being me. As a teacher, I get to form bonds with incredible kids who often teach me more than I teach them. Who are you?"

After this, Bill then proceeds to drop the fucking mic. Why was that so powerful? Because Bill was a man who had a story to tell, and that was exactly who I was going to be.

I had crazy stories filled with good days and bad ones. Provocative failures and critical success. Moments of self-righteousness where I should have held back. Times when the current was storming toward me, and I needed a helping hand. It was about time I gave someone else a helping hand. Rose someone else's spirits, proved they were capable of more than they could have ever imagined. Showed them all that there are battles to be fought but that the human spirit is powerful. That when you fail, time and time again, eventually, the ends will justify the means. The means might not be justified in the way that you thought they would, but not having the answers is what gives you a purpose.

The idea of chasing happiness will fail you. Your emotions will go to so many other places. Your mind will fill with anger, regret, sadness, trauma, fear, and to limit the brain to one way of thinking, to be "happy" is not only obstructive but also a complete waste.

So, feel it all, feel every single emotion possible because it's what makes you human.

Speaking of human, let's talk about something that happens to people every day. Peer pressure.

Some of us, unfortunately, will bend to peer pressure. Bend to fit the situation. It's OK to bend. We all must tolerate a certain degree of difference. But never stop being you. You're a quirky nerd? That's awesome, and that's exactly who you should be because that's you.

At one point in our lives, many of us want to be "cool," socially accepted, and fit in. We want to look "hot" or attractive, but it's all a distraction. They are expectations developed by societal values that are nothing but an illusion. What I believed in was not an illusion. What I wanted was real. I wanted to live. I wanted to gain my strength back, get back to school, and write a book. That is what was real to me. That was my dream. I went tooth and nail to chase a dream that was real. There were plenty of road signs along the way:

"In the next two miles, turn left and give up."

"Take the next exit and skip physical therapy."

That wasn't going to be my story. I refused to give up on myself, no matter the odds.

We may spend time with people who are not going to move us forward. It's a learning process, and in order to learn who is holding you back, you must experience being around non-productive people. How do you know? Ask yourself the following questions: *Is this person going to help me develop myself? Do they encourage me to be me?*

If they're trying to change who you are at your core, move on to more positive people. Learn from it and move forward. We all have our own personal struggles. But from my own experience, it's actually not success that makes you feel good about who you currently are. It's pushing yourself through difficult situations and coming out feeling prideful. That's what made me feel good.

I felt fantastic walking home in the freezing Canadian weather after a two-hour workout. It's not like I won a ton of money or was praised by others.

Nope, braving the cold and pushing my comfort zone was what made me feel electrified about being me.

And that's who I wanted to be. Me. So I called my high school leadership teacher Mr. Yonge, and he thought me sharing my story with his classes would be an incredible idea.

The planning began. I spent about two to three hours per day working on my story. Recalling facts, talking out loud, and designing the presentation in a way that I could effectively tell my story while simultaneously hitting as many emotional beats as possible. It was hard to dive into the past that felt so unreal but had taken place only months ago.

Day after day, I kept going. Knowledge of experience was about to overflow in my pitcher, and it was about time

I poured it into other people's cups. Share with people the hardship, the blood, sweat, and tears, and maybe they could find elements in my story to make a breakthrough in their own lives.

It was hard work, but if I could give one out of those eighty kids a new perspective, I had done my job.

What was so surprising about talking and putting my thoughts to paper was how therapeutic it was. It was one hundred percent me. Zero hiding.

Snow kept falling, and I kept gaining my strength. Slow as it was, steps were being taken. Moving forward, I was, and that I would continue to do.

I was pumped. Ready to show these kids that anything was possible. That the best motivational speakers are the ones who tell you, you can't achieve your dreams.

The week before, I was pulling the final pieces together. What once was scraps of paper now presented a story. I was so happy to still be here. Nervous as I was, it felt right. Time to go kick some ass and take some names. Well, maybe let's not do that; I don't want to get arrested.

My estimated run time was about forty minutes, give or take.

The day arrived, the sun rose, and I woke up excited, ready to rock and eventually roll out of bed.

I had made so much progress, and I believed in my ideas but was flexible to still think outside the box. Skinny as I was, I was a force to be reckoned with. That day my goal was to be a battery of emotion, sending currents of motivation and inspiration to everyone present with me in that room, to be a provider of such a rare resource (emotion).

I wanted to shake things up for the audience in a way they had never seen before. That day I would be a teacher. And as a teacher, I wanted to guide people to their own conclusions and, thus, their own idea of what the truth was to them.

I wanted to provide what was missing. Focus on legitimate, real tactics that I used to fight for my life. There are three basic components to the story I called The Girl, The Boat, And The Dragon. As the Boat and the Dragon are more relevant to the concepts I want to layout, those will be the ones we will be covering.

THE BOAT

MANY MOMENTS OF YOUR LIFE WILL HOLD SOME FORM OF STRUGGLE. You may not realize it, but there are periods of time where you are in turmoil, whether you accept it or not. The man or woman that does nothing every day and feels hopeless struggles because they don't act, sitting in despair, their mind continues to exaggerate fears to the point of no return. After they're knocked down, they stay down and come up with a Christmas list of reasons for why they can't get up.

For a while, I used cancer as an excuse for why I couldn't achieve my goals. I had nerve damage that decreased my strength and a crooked nose that made me feel unattractive. Man, was I good at it, creating excuses for why I couldn't become what I really wanted to be.

The winds that torment you and rock your boat are only made worse by you. You feel vulnerable like there is nothing you can do to land safely ashore.

I'm here to let you know there is no such thing as "the promised land" where everything is going to be perfect. Your boat will capsize, and the world will throw knives of current and cyclones to engulf you and your goals. You will continually be disappointed if you show up time and time again, expecting that the world will treat you nicely. The world's one job is to test you, flip your boat over, and throw challenge after challenge at you.

Let me tell you what your job is. Flip the boat back over, get back in, and start paddling. There is no engine, no motor to rely on because the engine and motor are you. Waves will come crashing, lightning will flash across the sky, but you must paddle. Even when you feel hopeless, you must paddle. If you want it, whatever that IT is, nothing will stop you. No peer pressure, no man, no woman, nothing will stop you. The forces of the world around you will continue to pound at you, whispering your greatest fears and worries. It's your job to get creative. Your paddle will break, and your boat may start to submerge below the surface.

As a human being, your mind is a powerful thing. People will be sitting at islands along the way, feeling comfortable, settling for "ordinary," but that ain't you. There will be obstacles and barriers that will make it seem impossible. You may feel ordinary, like you have zero passion. But we all have dreams and passions. It takes patience and trial and error. And it can be so frustrating to feel stuck.

I got so used to doing nothing, but everything changed when I started doing something about the nothing around me.

Many of us get hurt and run away from the pain. Nothing significant in your life will be accomplished without a dose of pain. There is beauty, but if you want it, you're going to have to be willing to make sacrifices. I had to sacrifice time wasted procrastinating and instead use that wasted time to improve myself. Because that's what I needed to do, I needed to take care of myself.

The storm is brewing above us all; it's raging, building up, unfathomable to our senses. It's scary to hear the storm scream that "we aren't good enough." That we are "destined to fail."

Today, maybe you aren't good enough. Today, maybe you did fail. But tomorrow is another day, another opportunity to put the gloves on and come out swinging.

Is it worth it? If you are even asking that question, you need to take a step forward and start taking action in your life.

Every day, I had to fight for small increments of improvement. It wasn't going to be a home run. But to take on the marathon that is life, to say, "I was dealt a shitty hand, but I'm all in." That's not just heroic. That's inspiring.

So, go out there, tiger. Go out with your retractable claws, but never retract. You are a beast. Yes, I'm talking about YOU. You just don't know it yet. So, what are you waiting for? The perfect moment? The inspirational calling? The numbers on your ticket to match up? Don't wait for the lottery. Stop rowing your boat towards millionaire island. Stop looking for what is already inside of you. You're already a millionaire. You just never had the courage to invest in yourself.

I wanted my life to go back to the way it was. I wanted a "big win." I dreamed of winning a free vacation, paddling my boat to shore, where I didn't have to worry about cancer anymore.

Invest in you. Read books, apply the knowledge gained from those books, and use it every single day you live and breathe. Hold back your wallets and ask yourself, will this benefit my long-term game?

It's totally acceptable to go out to the bar, get plastered, and have a good time while you're in your twenties. But I challenge you to limit yourself and establish self-control. Go out and party. Just don't do it excessively.

"Oh, Chris, just one more drink!" Seriously? How many times have you said that now? A lot, too much in fact. That one sentence adds up in dollars. First to the tens, then the twenties, and people eventually find themselves in a hole so deep they can't find a way out, and they wonder how they got there. That's where the victim card comes in, "Why me?" Why you? Are you kidding me? That's the best answer you got? I'll tell you why. You never learned where to take your boat. When the going got tough, you paddled back and stayed at party island instead of hustling. You bought 300-dollar shoes, when you could have spent sixty.

So, go out there and face the challenges life throws at you. Paddle towards the storm. The old saying rings true. The grass is always greener on the other side. The question is, do you want it bad enough?

If you want debt, a meaningless life, and empty memories, by all means, go for it. Nobody's gonna stop you.

But twenty years later, when Dave's kids ask if he is proud of who he's become. Dave may say, "Yes, Suzy, I am." But Dave truly wishes he had made better choices. But Dave, it's never over. No matter how old, no matter how late. There is always an opportunity to better yourself and the ones around you. So, don't be too hard on yourself, Dave. We all make mistakes.

Jump in the boat, and paddle-like your life depends on it because it does.

On that warm summer's day of June 2018. That is exactly what I told those kids.

THE DRAGON

THE DRAGON TOWERED OVER ITS MOUNTAINOUS PILE OF GOLD. His ruby-like scales glowed brightly, along with the fire-like eyes that burned with ferocity. Silence, then a roar that shook the room like an earthquake. The gold around us bounced as the sound sent vibrations through our spines. Outside the cave, my breath had been mist floating away like a lost thought, no longer tangible.

Mason's eyes met Fynne's, then Jane's, and then they ran. From one pillar to the next. The fiery flames came out in a gust, licking at the air around them. One fraction of a second too late, and the three would have been toast. The dragon spread its wings, and a whirlwind of air sent gold flying throughout the room. Mason had never seen anything quite like it. The beast had killed and hoarded for years. Hundreds of thousands of innocent lives had been taken. It was time to end him. It was time to take him down.

For centuries they had called him Draak. No longer would he continue to rule. Today he would become a tale of what once was. It was time to slay the dragon.

Mason turned the corner and his eyes locked with the beast.

We all have our own demons, our own dragon to slay. Many of us will run away when our dragon confronts us. Why try? It's impossible. The odds are so slim.

Let me ask you this when Martin Luther King decided he was going to stand up for equality, did he accept slim odds and live with them? No, that man lived in the present moment, whether that moment was hell or heavenly.

With cancer, I often lived in the hell. There was always an opportunity to give in, throw in the towel and say, "I quit." But cancer wasn't going to get the best of me. There are millions of unwinnable battles that are won. The chances may look slim, but by quitting, you're only guaranteeing your failure.

No matter how bad you have it, always remember that a one-in-a-million shot is better than no shot at all. Take the shot, bleed the belief that you have buried so deep inside yourself. Grab the spade and dig. I don't care how much you have to dig. Dig deep, and when you hit steel, grab a drill and tear it apart. Take the hits, fight like hell, and face that dragon upon the mountain of gold.

Become a slayer of your own dragon. Face the fear. You are ready to face your fears. Face the overweight version of you. That's you now, but that doesn't have to be you tomorrow. Wake up early if you have to. Feeling tired? Take the needed rest and come back. You scared? You should be. What's scarier than the dragon upon the mountain of gold? The version of you that never came to be.

No one is going to inspire you more than you. Aspire to be the hero that slays his or her own dragon, that takes all the riches from the beast's chambers. Share that experience and wealth with the world. Because once you prove that you are an unstoppable force, the rest of us will see that it's possible to crush our own fears and rise above the limitations that we've conjured up in our own heads. And your mind will continue to conjure up fear if you sit there expecting to change. The Earth is about to complete another rotation, and you still haven't done anything.

What do you want written on your gravestone? My name was Dan. I hooked up with chicks at bars, never learned which ones cared about me, got drunk every day, and worked a job I hated.

Or my name was Dan. Even when I failed, I brushed off the dirt and kept going. I faced every single obstacle in my path and did my best to learn from every encounter. I laughed, cried, won, and failed. I'm proud to say I lived the best fucking life I could.

We all have challenges, but never, ever let them consume you. You must consume them, and that's an order.

Start planning, get creative, map out how you are going to slay your dragon. "But Chris, my plan sucks! It's so lame!" A plan soaking in the waters of mediocrity is better than no plan at all. Adjust yourself to the notion of being flawed. I got used to that when I came out of surgery with a crooked nose. People gave me looks.

Some of fear, others of curiosity. Others notably saw it as a flaw. It sucked and still sucks, but that doesn't stop me from meeting new people or going to the gym. I love life and want to make the most of it.

It's time to buckle in and commit to tackling what scares you. If you're living a "safe" or "comfortable" life, that's part of the problem. The reason why nothing extraordinary is happening is because by accepting safety, you're also taking along a very predictable life with no risk or challenge along with it.

Step onto the fiery flames the dragon has set out in front of you. You will not only gain respect from others but also from yourself. That shit is key. Nobody is going to respect you if you don't first take the time to discover what makes you so fucking awesome.

You may think you're not talented enough. That you are incapable of greatness. But there is no secret sauce for greatness. More talented people might have it easier, but they aren't guaranteed success. Take action, big or small, do it. The hardest step to take is always the first one.

Taking the first step is the beginning of a whole new journey to unraveling who that person is. What makes it scary is you don't know who that person is...yet. They could be anyone. Many of us don't fear who we are. We fear who we could become. That new person may come with an entirely new motherboard that runs it, and it's scary as hell to accept, "Yeah, I might need to change."

Changing yourself physically or mentally is tough. If it was easy, everybody would be changing to improve their lives and ways of living.

Step one. Identify what you want. That might be a hiking trip through the mountains near Seattle. Elevate yourself thousands of feet. Breathe in the success of achieving that goal. Inhale the humid air and continue crushing goals.

What if you don't know what you want? My answer to you is to ask questions and take initiative. You shouldn't have the expectation that the answers will be given to you on a platter cooked and ready for the taking. Sometimes you're going to have to take your GPS out and search for that shit. You might trip over a rock and get completely lost. But through all of that, you come out a tougher person, with a deeper understanding of yourself and the obstacles you have overcome along the way.

My aunt Karen got lost in a forest once. She took a course on how to survive, and well, I guess you could say that things didn't go as planned, and she got lost. She told me the story in dark and dramatic tones. That did not stop me from laughing my ass off. I was a complete jerk for laughing, but damn, was that shit funny. And she laughed too. It's a part of life. In the next one hundred years of your life, you are going to get lost in some way, shape, or form. I just hope, for your sake, you don't get lost in a forest. [9]

All of us will get lost. We may not get lost in a forest, but we will get lost. I'm still lost. Hell, there is no three-step guide to reintegrating yourself back into society after stage four cancer. I fucking wish. If you happen to find a guide, send that shit my way, but until then, I'll continue the struggle.

What I wanted was to get back to a "normal" twenty-year-old life. It is not easy, but that does not stop me from trying. I continue working out, writing, and catching up with family and friends. I have moments where I feel like things aren't working out, but that's just an inevitable part of life.

That brings us to step two—lace-up. Put on the gloves

9   Thank you to my Aunt Karen for giving permission to talk about you. Your support meant the world.

and get ready to get hit. Let those hits sink in and acknowledge the pain. But never let it stop you. Chase what your heart desperately needs, what your spirit thirsts for.

Many give in and fall into line with what others think they should be. The strongest of us push other's negativity out of the way and refuse to give up on ourselves. Fight your way back, punch through the pain. Let the others talk, challenge ideas, stand up for you because you deserve that.

Take the hits but always keep moving forward. You do those two things, and you're already ahead of the game.

It's your time to do good; it's your time to fail, so go do it. Because many people are a waste of your damn time. Stop being "Mr. Nice Guy." It's important to be polite, but don't become a "people pleaser."

You will never achieve your goals if you are too busy trying to make other people happy. Find a symbiotic relationship. That's right, I just took you back to science class for a brief moment. But seriously, search for people that encourage you to be the best version of you and vice versa. Once you do find them, your life, while still filled with challenge and struggle, will also have close friends to keep you going and run the marathon with you in times of need.

Step three, victory. You did it. After so much struggle, pain, and sacrifice, here you are. You will feel relief, exhaustion, and a fuck ton of pride. To go mile after mile and continue running with all the pain, all the lactic acid that builds up and torments you. That is exceptional.

When I heard those words. "Chris, we saw no trace of remaining cancer. He was able to remove every last bit. You're cancer-free." I can't describe how happy I was. This meant everything to me. My life wasn't over. I could continue writing, working out, and spending time with my family and friends. Here's the mistake you don't want to make. All the riches you discovered need to be shared with the people you love.

Giving often feels better than receiving. There is nothing more special than when a loved one opens a Christmas present and starts crying out of love. You can't put a price on that moment. Moments define us, and they can show how loving we can be to one another. Take in those moments like a sponge, absorb all the love and laughter gained in that moment. Life is filled with extravagant moments of grief and despair. Learn to live in the good moments while you can. Those loving people in your life won't be around forever, and neither will you.

Those riches you gain from your dragon must be shared. You only get what you give. Start giving.

BEING A LEADER

CRAZY SHIT IS GONNA GO DOWN. That's right, wild stuff. That person you went to high school with is about to become a parent at fifteen. You will see someone get so drunk that they start to believe that they are Moses. And that it's their destiny to build bridges to sacred sanctuaries for the people who need the guiding life.

Life is bound to get crazy, and there will be things that happen that make you freeze up. Your arms will just seem to stop working right then and there, and that will be it. And when you look back upon that moment and try to pick it apart, it will be nothing but a blur, a lost memory floating in the empty space of your mind.

The event will feel like a movie. It was like you were there but not truly there.

All you will remember will be the flashing lights and the sirens when they came. Our brains do a fantastic job of protecting us. They bury our troubles deep down where they will never be able to hurt us.

These troubles can stay down there for a long time, and while we may feel safe, once they present themselves, it all can become unbearable. That's when the understanding comes into play, where the pieces click and form fear in our heads. That moment where you saw someone get shot becomes a reality after the terror had been buried for so long. That memory of when you were rejected socially and made fun of comes up to bite you in the ass.

When that thing does surface, whatever it is, it will feel like a shockwave. You will attempt to explain the situation to others, and they will nod their heads and say, "Ya, I totally get it." But they won't. You wish they understood what it feels like to see something unbearable, but we often stay in our own safe fishbowl to thrive in. One where we don't have to adjust, where we can live as close to a perfect world as we can without heartbreak or consequence.

Sounds amazing, doesn't it? Smash the fishbowl. It's an ocean out there. You have to fight for resources. [10]

At this moment, in my local area, there are thousands of people with degrees that are unemployed. I bet you that many of these people envisioned a steady job and life with a degree in their hands.

It doesn't matter how many times you've practised or run the drills through your mind. It will never be enough. We don't study to increase our certainty. We study to decrease our uncertainty.

No other species craves answers more than us. And It's gotten us far. We no longer have to throw our shit out of the window. Thank God for that. Now, with one simple push of a button, we can make our shit and our problems disappear without a trace.

---

10 Thanks to my aunt Mari-Angela for giving me the go on this story. Much love.

About a month ago, I witnessed an accident that was absolutely bonkers. Yep, I just dropped the "B" word bitches. But this accident came out of nowhere. I guess that makes sense because no accident is predictable.

It was cold out. I mean freezing. You think it gets cold in Houston in the winter? I will take your ten-degree winter over our minus twenty-one in a heartbeat. You call me, and we will arrange that shit pronto. Your wish is my command.

I saw someone get hit by a car. They were walking next to me, to my left, about fifteen feet behind me. I coincidentally had turned my head the moment it had happened. Their body flipped and soared through the air like a fighter jet.

I'll never forget how fast my aunt Mari-Angela took action. Zero fucking hesitation. She immediately dived into the situation. Other people did too, but out of panic. They picked the victim up after they had been hit. Never do that. It was awesome that these people cared, but that was not the right move. My aunt screamed for them to stop, but the panic had taken them over. My aunt was able to act logically in a chaotic environment. When everyone else was losing their minds, my aunt remained calm, cool, and collected. That scenario you hear about when people ask for the 9-1-1 number after they had just said 9-1-1. I can confirm, as a witness, that it is true.

But what makes a person have the courage to operate through the pain and chaos? Trauma.

From my own experience, trauma teaches you to take action instead of waiting around for the hand of God to save you. Why wait when you can become the saving hand? Why wait when you can become the leader?

But what if I go for it and fail? Yeah. What's worse than trying and failing? Doing nothing and wondering what if I had made the effort? Nothing hurts more than the 'what ifs' and 'what could have beens.' Don't fight the moments that come across you. Run with them. It's scary as hell because you're so used to waiting it out.

When I was in ICU, I was surrounded by people who were willing to lead. They were there in a flash and gave me nothing but the best. To have others drop what they're doing at a moment's notice for you makes you feel loved and appreciated. And during those hellish moments, seeing one of the nurses smile at me like I was the best man in the world made me feel so loved.

They didn't have to work in Neuro ICU. There were plenty of other career paths along the way. But they chose the hard path. I could not have done it without you. You laughed with me when I needed it most, and you talked with me when I needed to feel like a human being.

It's funny how the things we really need get lost in unnecessary meandering down a curving river that is leading us nowhere. But it's a path regardless, so we stay put and continue sipping our exotic drinks, watching all the sights pass us without ever experiencing or learning anything.

A man named Damon had travelled along a river in a remote forest far to the east, in search of answers from a monk. Damon journeyed on a boat was loaded with great wines and whiskeys. And so, Damon drank. And once one bottle went dry, he picked up a second. By the time Damon had arrived, he could barely stand up. He stood up, belched, and made his way over to the monk's temple. And at the end of the journey, there was reason why Damon stood in front of the wise monk, drunk with all the wrong answers.

The monk had told Damon to make the journey and to tell him what he had seen along the way. There were many things to be seen.

Starved people gathering in the shallows. Drug-infested societies, raging with the cries of lost souls in the mountainous regions of the dense jungle. The clouds flowed low and heavy throughout the hills. Shabby houses sat on the shore. Fisherman desperately hunted for the next catch, but Damon saw none of it.

Once Damon had arrived with no answer, the Monk sent him back to watch again. However, this time was different. Damon was no longer too ignorant to drink from the bottle, but instead, he was now able to pay enough attention to what was going on around him.

The young men and women skinny as rails were now clearer to Damon than they had ever been before. The heavy bags forming under the fishermen's eyes stared back into Damon's. But there was something different among it all.

A man was sitting calmly upon a stone pyre. His face was relaxed, though his arms rested in a meditative fashion, crossed in front of him. His chest displayed a tattoo of a winged horse. Calligraphy patterns were etched in ink across his arms.

The Monk shouted at two boys fighting one another. He encouraged them fiercely, belting out a steady, controlled flow of commands. "Keep going!" The Monk encouraged. "Cut him down!"

The Monk's mission was to give lost souls a purpose. His

guidelines kept the children from the drugs and negativity that surrounded them. The law would not forgive these kids, many of their own families would never forgive them, but the Monk would and did. The Monk wanted to lead a new way.

Many people in the tribes had fallen victim to the drug culture within the forest, along with the disease. The tribe spoke a different tongue and dressed in a different manner compared to an outsider.

The Monk trained the children hard and gave them discipline. The children struggled, and the training was brutal. Their shins began to feel fragile from kicking and receiving blows. But the training continued, and slowly but surely, their bones turned into steel. And while the journey was treacherous, it now provided the students with the means, motivation, and courage to keep struggling.

The journey eventually came to an end. Damon knelt down in front of the wise man who asked him, "What have you learned?"

"I've learned to serve."

"Serve whom?" The wise man beckoned.

"Serve those who are dreaming of reaching impossible heights."

The wise man smiled and gave a subtle nod. "Good, now it is your turn to lead the way."

FEAR

THE CANCER WAS GONE, BUT EVERYTHING HAD CHANGED. My brain was damaged and healing, and most people I came across had their own routines. And I was scared.

After all that had happened, I felt fear of so many things. Social skills had become outdated when not used in the field. Plus, after nearly dying, I found it impossible to trust people due to the fear of being hurt even more than I already was.

I lived many days in the shadows, not wanting to be scorched in the light. I often listened to music so I could escape. I put on the headphones and went for a walk. I didn't know what else to do. I was scared shitless.

What if I remained crippled from the treatments? What if nobody would hire me ever again? Because why would they? When another, more capable, person could stand in my place?

Questions bounced around my head, rattling hisses and baring their teeth. And as I saw other people going to parties and forming new bonds with others, it started to make me feel like an outcast.

I did not want to feel alone, but I did. I felt cheated. I had the shot lined up, but it turns out the gun was never loaded in the first place.

Fear created a constant worry. It seemed like things were working out for others, but why not me? Why could I not have the answers given? I want the cheat sheet.

What was the point anymore? Wake up to a post-apocalyptic hell, rinse and repeat.

I walked to music in the rain with the rain beating down on me. Today a grey sky, tomorrow hopefully a blue.

One day Mumford and Sons, the next Foo Fighters.

At the time, I always walked where there would be no other people. I gave up on people at this point. They saw my bald head and skinny, frail body and looked away. They gave me looks of sorrow or fear. I was sick of people giving me those looks, so I walked where nobody could give them to me.

A memory of walking through the cold along the powerlines with a friend would come back to me. That was a memory from before my post-apocalyptic hell. Gosh, in that moment, all I had to complain about was the cold. I wish that's all I had to complain about now.

I wish I had someone to walk with. All my friends were understandably busy with school, tied down with responsibility. That didn't make the fear go away. If I were to remain in this state, who would have the time for me? My answer at the time was nobody.

The fear got the best of me, and I continued keeping to myself and away from others. I never wanted someone to look at me that way again, and if I hid away, nobody would ever have the chance. I did this for a while. The fear kept me at bay, but parts of it were necessary. In order to heal, sometimes, you do need to pull yourself away from everything.

Give yourself time to process.

If asked how I was doing, I responded, "good." Because telling people how I really felt would just turn me into emotional baggage that no one would ever want to be around.

Fear holds us back. Fear takes many forms. A spider lowering itself on a thin, wiry strand of web, a snake slithering through the sands or a shark swimming in the depths.

Fear was so prevalent when getting cancer treatment. The number of people struggling in the hospital. So desperate for a better tomorrow. The flashing lights of ambulances pulling in and out. The sirens wailing in the dead of night.

The mistake I made was I let the fear take control of me. I let it own who I was. I was scared. Fuck fear.

When it comes to fear, it can take control of us, and it can leave us completely paralyzed. We can get so wrapped up in fear that we become afraid of not just the shark swimming in the depths, but of how terrified that feeling of fear is to us. Fear will devour you if you let it.

We all get scared in our own little ways. We get scared when we're about to open up our test results, we become nervous on our way to a job interview, and we shake when we're about to ask out that person we're interested in. And the worst part of it all isn't the fear. No, the worst part is that the fear stops us from taking a chance on ourselves. It stops us from trying.

So, go do it. Open up that test and look at that mark. Get dressed and go to that interview because you're about to fucking nail it. And ask out that person you're interested in. Will you feel fear? Absolutely. But the fear is only worth five seconds of your time. Feel that fear for those five seconds and go do that thing you want to do. Because you know what? That thing might just happen. And who knows? It might even change your life.

That-5 second rule is huge. And I use it when fear comes across me.

One of my biggest struggles was how much I would overthink. My mind would just get too damn carried away. I'd get so caught up in all the what-ifs and all the things that could go wrong. I beat myself down when I should have been building myself up. I want you to do it. Let that fear in. Absorb that shit. Let it soak you from head to toe. Let it send shivers down your spine. Let it whisper in your ear. But never, ever, let it take control of you. It's only worth five seconds of your time and no more.

Fear is contagious, a disease. It stops us from becoming who we were always meant to be. It stops us from loving, living, and growing. Fear is a sickness, and when consumed by it, I felt lost. As if there was no way out. And the more I feared, the more I struggled to live.

I lived in fear for a year. Scared if I was ever going to live. Afraid that I would never have the opportunity to have children, get married, and have a family. It scared me so much. Fear took me over. I hated fear, but fear loved me. It grew stronger the weaker I got. Fear was a parasite leeching off me. Taking the life from me. Sucking the breath out from my chest. Fear is a cancer. But just like cancer, fear can be beaten. So, give the fear five seconds. And no more. Because you are bigger than your fears, never forget that.

I let that fear in. That negative shit that pulled me down

every single day. I let it in, and I spoke to it. Fear is only as real as we make it. It's a picture and nothing more. Look at that picture but never let the painting of fear define you. I believe I lived because I chose to face my fear. Faced the reality of the situation I was in. I never chose cancer. I never wanted to see the people I love cry next to me in a hospital bed. I never wanted to see anybody struggle for me. It hurt like hell. But it's better to hurt than to feel nothing at all. Everyone hurts. The fear, the fights, the losses. We all know it. And if we don't know it already, sadly, we will. On the other side of fear is everything. Love, friendship, and success.

> "Everything you've ever dreamed of is
> on the other side of fear."
> — Christopher Sean Stewart

All I ever wanted was to live and love. What separated me from love and life was a wall of fear. Face fear, and nothing can stop you. Face fear, and you won't regret it. And when fear comes back knocking at your door, face it again. The fear has it all wrong. Fear is a beast that thinks it is in control. But when push comes to shove, fear should be afraid of you. You, yes, you! Fear has no idea what you're capable of. Fear has no idea the ideas you have; fear doesn't have your vision. Own the fear and own every single second of your life. It's your life, and it's yours to live, so live the fuck out of it.

Do that thing you've always wanted to do! Give yourself permission. Just do it. And if it works out, great. If it doesn't, reassess and keep on keeping on. Apply for that university class you were hesitant about, join clubs and meet people. There will be failures along the way. Brush it off and move on. Because when you give fear more than five seconds, you're showing fear that it's worth your time. And it's not. Life is hard, but once you accept the fear, you'll start to see all the wealth on the other side. Fear should be scared shitless of you. If you're persistent and are always willing to learn, progress will be made.

We have hopes and dreams. We hope things will fall into place. We dream our dreams will become our realities.

We all can become self-conscious about who we are. And unfortunately, there are many people who feel unaccepted, unappreciated, and unloved. The harsh reality is most people don't have time for you. The sooner you realize that, the better.

I always tried my best to spare some time for other people.

People started sending me messages. Asking me how I dealt with it. The fear, the trauma. I will always offer a helping hand when I can. It's in my DNA. I wanted nothing more than to help the people entrusting me with their personal struggles. I realized at that moment how closed many people have become. Many are afraid to be who they really are. I locked away my problems, turned my back, and pretended that they were not there. There are others who lock away abuse and tragedy. They bury it away so deep that no one will ever find it, not even they, themselves. My tragedies are horrible. They bring back aches, pains, and I just wanted it to go away. Go away forever where it couldn't hurt my family anymore. I got sick of hurting, but I always kept the promise I made to my dad. No matter how hard it got, I would never give up on myself.

It's not our tragedies that define us, but how we come back

from them. I'm not just some kid who was diagnosed with cancer. I'm a survivor and a warrior. So, don't let the fear define you. Let the victories and the strength define who you are.

We all get knocked down. It's how we get up that defines us. It's a part of life. Puzzles get messy, glass gets broken, people become fractured. We ourselves become fractured.

I want you to lose yourself. And after you lose yourself, I want you to find yourself all over again. Fall in love with who you are. You're fucking incredible and never forget that. Not for a second. Give yourself credit and stop being so damn hard on yourself. Fear may define you for a moment, but you're more than a moment. You're a legacy waiting to be written. You're a miracle. The things you're capable of, and the people that love you. The people who have yet to love you. The laughs you'll have. It's all there, right in front of you. You just have to go get it.

Everything that makes life worth living is on the other side of fear. So, do it. Get up at 5:00 a.m. and hustle. Get out there and chase that career that you've always dreamed of. Go do it because you have an amazing opportunity to live an incredible life with extraordinary people.

I got so caught up in the fear. "I'm not smart enough. I'm too skinny. I'm not the right man for the job." I could continue letting fear dictate my actions, or I could say, "Fuck it!" "Bring it on fear!" Sure, there would be bumps along the road. There would be pain, regret, and loss. But you have a choice. Face the fear now and deal with that along the way. Or fear every single day for the rest of your life.

Live every day like it's your last. It damn well could be. I never saw stage 4 cancer coming. Hell, nobody did. One of the beautiful parts of life is we don't know what's around the corner. It may be scary but also beautiful. The northern lights flashing up on a night hike, making the person you love smile. Or getting drunk on the porch with your best friends.

You can't give in to the fear. Take a chance on you. Believe in you. It will be uncomfortable. There will be countless moments of struggle and frustration. Where all you're thinking is, *what the fuck am I doing?* The fear will pull in like a tide. But just like the tide, fear comes and goes in waves. It never stays. It only visits. Give the tide those five seconds. Feel the sand below your feet and the water slip between your toes. And watch the tide pull away.

The tide will always be there taunting you, trying to convince you that you're not good enough, that you're incapable. If every person on the planet thought that they were incapable of greatness, where would we be? Nowhere. The biggest gamble you have to make in life is on yourself. Once you face the fear and go all in, that is when you'll truly start living life. The fear will never go away. But there are many other things that won't go away either. Friendship, family, and streaming. It will all be waiting for you to lend a helping hand when the fear starts to sink in. Fear will sink in but never, ever let fear sink you.

The rocky waters of fear surround us. It's our job to do our best to navigate those waters. We're scared to take the initiative. We're scared to take responsibility when the odds seem so low. Hell, I know. I know it's scary to be you. It's hard. When I walked with Paul, my chemo pole, throughout those hospital walls, I was afraid. But when I saw my family, it gave me strength, it gave me courage, and the fear went away. I didn't feel the fear. All I felt was my mother's and father's arms wrapped around me.

My dad often worked, the relaxing sound of the keys clicking as he tapped away. It came and went like rain. It was peaceful. I tried to fight the sleep, but I eventually would drift off, dreaming about being anywhere but here in the hospital.

Three hours later, I would wake up to see my mother's face. She always believed in me, and that gave me comfort. My aunt Karen often came in at the same time. T.V was often a hot topic of conversation. It helped keep me distracted from all the things going wrong. We also spent time predicting which characters would die next and who would gain the upper hand. We ordered Chinese food, sandwiches, or burgers. Whatever my stomach could handle at that moment.

I often would take a lap around the third floor with my dad (and Paul the IV pole). We walked slowly. *One foot in front of the other,* I thought. *One foot in front of the other. One, two, one, two, one, two.*

I would always try to smile at the nurses as they passed. I wanted to show them I was a fighter, that I wouldn't let the fear rule my life, that I was a winner. My gut told me that I was going to win. No matter what anybody said, my heart and spirit were too big to be crushed. I knew there were going to be ups and downs. I knew fear would return, but that's what my family was there for.

Fear can disable us in many ways. Fear can stop us from believing in ourselves, achieving our goals, and ultimately, fear can prevent us from pursuing the life that we really want.

I wasn't going to let fear kill my dream of living again. Life can be painfully unpredictable, and it moves in mysterious ways. And at times, you will feel like giving up. You will feel like throwing in the towel and calling it quits. The world is too big, and you just feel so small. That's the fear talking.

It's your time to put the pedal to the metal. We see other's success, other's victories, and we can get discouraged. "Why isn't that me? I want that promotion! I want that car!" But here's the thing, you got it all backwards. Your value as a human being is not measured by the car you drive, the amount of money you have, or the number of followers you have. No, it starts with you. It starts with waking up and facing the fear. Accepting that you're not perfect, dealing with loss, getting punished for mistakes but refusing to let the fear take control. It starts with you. Not the fancy car or big house. That's such a poor value system. You're more than a fancy piece of metal on wheels. You're thirty to forty trillion cells[11] of badassery.

We get so caught up in social and financial status based on what we own. We shouldn't fight for wealth and riches, but for wealth of love and laughter. A sports car is half a million dollars. My family is worth more than any number you could throw at me. We need money to survive. But without love, we're scared and alone. Without love, we're nothing.

But you are more than nothing. The day you realize that and start facing fear is the day you will be reborn. Fuck fear.

---

11 Eva Bianconi et al., "An estimation of the number of cells in the human body," Annal of Human Biology 40, no. 6 (November 2013): 463-471, https://doi.org/10.3109/03014460.2013.807878.

CHAOS

MY OLD HIGH SCHOOL WAS RUNNING ANOTHER BIKEATHON. The goal was half a million. I had my doubts, but I did still think Mr. Yonge and his leadership class could do it.

Organizing the event was a frenzy of chaos. The amount of paperwork and team effort is quite astounding. From my own experience, there are still some people who didn't contribute much. But for the most part, a group effort was present.

When the day came, I went in with my guard up high. I still felt very cautious and walked the school only talking with people I felt were genuine. Now, you might be wondering, *why immerse yourself in the chaos after all the fear?* Well, you will eventually be too fed up with waiting, or you will start to care about something, or both. Not only was I sick of being scared, but I believed in the work that Mr. Yonge did. I'll never forget my first class with Mr. Yonge in grade ten.

He burst into the room, where forty of us sat, and proceeded to jump on a table singing *Do you hear the people sing* from *Les Misérables.*[12] He sang the song with energy

---

12 Permission granted from Tom Yonge and Mr. Van Ginhoven to talk about this experience as well as my experience at Scona, Verbal and email permission provided.

and charisma. He even got in each of our faces, making one person laugh and the next filled with shock.

What a way to make a first impression. Imagine entering your first day at work to find the boss laying it all out on the floor. I'm talking about the sickest moves you've ever seen.

Mr. Yonge (while many people were wondering what the hell they had signed up for) was able to captivate an audience and hold their attention with a two-and-a-half-minute spur of chaos. Some classes were boring throughout school, and while people had their own ideas of what leadership was, I rarely ever associate the word "boring" with it.

People love making sense of the chaos, whether they realize it or not. That's what made leadership fun and refreshing to me.

Immersing myself into the situation was hard. Many of the people around me knew what had happened to me, and it made my mind spin. It made me glance over my shoulder, thinking to myself, *I wonder what they're thinking of me?*

My doctor had put me on a medication to help with the cold hands and feet (which have fortunately gotten better). I felt antsy and on edge, and my anxiety post-cancer made me a happy-go-lucky kind of guy. Happy for a couple of days, then out of nowhere, I would feel down. We all get sad, but depression after cancer at eighteen?! That's on a whole other level.

Because of this, I often would feel lost or unwanted in situations. Especially being back at school. It only seems like yesterday that I had been in a positive form of chaos. A chaos with school assignments, a chaos where my life wasn't on the line. This new post-cancer chaos had no sense of order to it at all. All these people that had no clue what life may hold in store for them. All the looks of curiosity and the numerous sets of dodgy eyes that came with them—what do I do with that type of chaos?

Regardless, I did what Mr. Yonge said to our class years ago. To push myself out of my comfort zone. I felt so uncomfortable, but when I look back at it, I feel proud. Leadership class had given me faith that there were good people and good causes in the world. And I looked forward to coming to school to do just that: to push myself and try to make the world a better place.

But in my second year of high school, I lost faith in the prospect of good people. And when someone gets hurt, their guard automatically rises to prevent getting hurt in the same way again. So, I stayed away from the chaos that other people had to offer. I was healing. Instead, I went to school, kickboxed at night, ran the power lines, and did everything in my power to avoid the unpredictable nature of people. I could never be shot if I was never present in the crosshairs.

Kickboxing was its own special form of chaos. It was a vicious chess game that came with a mental and physical cost. It hurts to get hit. The only thing that relieved the pain was a warm shower and a deep sleep. I listened to those who taught me and gave my best. Sometimes, my best wasn't enough, and sometimes it was. I did it because it made me feel stronger. Kickboxing showed me that I could come back, time and time again, and fight with spirit, grit, and determination.

One night, back before cancer chaos, I got punched in the face really hard and came home with a black eye. I went to school the next day. People didn't know I kickboxed, so I guess they just thought I got into trouble. Whatever they thought, it didn't matter. It was badass—period.

This time around, at my return to Scona (post-diagnosis), I didn't have a black eye, but a crooked nose, and my face looked puffy from inflammation. I judged myself for the way that I looked. Fortunately, I will be getting cosmetic surgery to straighten things out. But for now I must continue to deal with it.

We all judge ourselves. The first thing that you see in the morning every day will often be you. Having so many mirrors can be a bit of a problem. Our brains already have too much going on, and having to look back at my new face that was me—but wasn't me—was hard.

We can't control the way we feel. We can hold ourselves back from arguing when we're angry, but we're still angry. We can pretend to smile when we feel down, but we're still sad. It's not our fault for feeling emotions. It's a part of who we are.

I felt many negative emotions throughout my fight against cancer. A chaotic spur of negative nonsense went throughout my head at times, and it was easy to let it run when I had a total lack of purpose at the time.

My job at the time was to heal.

When your life purpose is to sit there and wait, man, does it suck. I was sitting and waiting for my life to change. I was a dude who took initiative. And when everyone around me was telling me that "it would take time." I can't lie to you; it was extremely gut-wrenching.

Most of the people I knew had some kind of purpose.

A family to raise, nights of drinking, studying to do. Big or small, they had some sort of chaos to immerse themselves in. Chaos is stressful, feels exhausting, and can make you, at times, hate your life. But I would take chaos with a purpose over waiting, any day.

So be grateful for what you have. Our lives are crazy, and life sure isn't always fair. But one of the biggest mistakes you can make is getting so lost in the chaos that you begin to take the important stuff for granted.

Chaos led to pain.

PAIN

GOING BACK TO AND VISITING SCONA WAS NECESSARY. The trip led me to a lot of discovery not only about myself, but about others as well. I had changed dramatically, but the people around me had not.

Many cancer survivors I have met have said that the hardship they survived gave them a better appreciation for life and for those they loved. Each person had their unique set of experiences, but other survivors could relate to these stories through their similarities to their own—they'd been there—they knew. What made the trip to the school so painful was that I had just come out of my own war, but there was no one who could empathize with me.

I will forever be grateful to those who showed up and supported me—those who made me feel like a million bucks when I felt like nothing at all. The thing is, none of my family and friends understood what it felt like to have your life flipped in a split second, to have people treat you differently after an altered appearance. Nobody understood the amount of pain I went through. They could guess what it was like, but that's just the thing. Sympathy and empathy are two completely different leagues. Sympathy is the little league: a bunch of kids screaming, celebrating "the big win," and watching cartoons on the weekends. Empathy is a whole other ball game. Welcome to the major league, folks. Buckle up this is going to be one hell of a ride.

We've all seen the example I'm about to layout, so let me lay this out for you. Two dudes become homies overnight because they both hate the same thing. Brad brings up how much he hates the Mallar Knights. He just hates everything about them. He's a true Falcons fan through and through.

Jeff, while he isn't a Falcons fan (because he was born in Caper) does wholeheartedly agree about hating on the Knights. Boom, a bromance emerges more powerful than any magic ever seen. There's nothing that can break these two dudes apart.

We can sometimes bond over hate. Because when another person in the room passionately hates the same thing as you, a light bulb goes off, and before you can even think, you are hopping on the hate train. And often, jumping on the hate train is easier. It can, in many cases, be the less painful thing to do, as you're not challenging the opinion of others.

There is a choice that must be made when deciding who you want to be. This choice can be made right now at this very moment. The question is, are you a winner or a loser? If you really are a winner, you will challenge the pain that will come at you every day for the rest of your life. You will accept that people will tell you "no" or that you are "incapable," and you will use that as motivation. You will recognize that the people who tell you these things fell victim to the pain around them and fell into line with the proposed perception that others conceived of them.

Don't get stuck on other's preconceived notions of you. You decide who you want to be, period. Don't let them get the best of you, not even for a second. The pains in your life can be awful, where day after day passes and you feel so lost, and that feeling of loss never seems to go away. There is no answer to life. There is no saving grace out there because the saving grace is you.

I save my pain and suffering by bettering myself—doing brain therapy after the trauma, writing music, going for runs, spending time with the people who matter, and feeling sick after eating too many nachos.

Living already comes with enough pain. Make it easier on yourself. See your value as an amazing person. Ask out people who make the pains that come with life more bearable. You should never have to endure pain alone; endure and prosper with the ones who love you. That's the real shit.

When I returned to Scona, I thought that I could get back the feeling that leadership class and Mr. Yonge had given me in the first place. The problem was that it had been a different time, a different life. I was licking my war wounds by trying to live a life that had been gone for months. It was hard to accept that my old life was gone. But I had no choice. I had to move on. I had to let go.

Letting go of what you love is hard. I wanted nothing more than to continue living the life I had been living. I realized that dreaming about the good old days wasn't living. It was dying. I was returning to those memories to avoid how much pain my present held.

I decided to find a way to cope with the pain. I talked with my family about my struggles, and that helped.

Opening up the floodgates and relieving the built-up pressure is always good.

What helped treat my pains will seem counter-intuitive, but I treated my pain with more pain. Pushing myself at the gym, the reminder of how physically weak I was, was the most effective way to deal with the pain of living post-cancer. I came back home feeling tired and sweaty, replacing life pain with the pain of pride and progress. It's not a perfect solution, but imperfection is what makes us human. And boy, did I ever feel human. I felt it all: the sore back, dry throat, cold winter winds, hot summer air.

Enjoy the car you have to drive and the options you have in your life; Love it, and never forget how lucky you are. While you don't have everything, you sure as hell have enough.

I would love to have my license back, which had been taken away due to a blind spot resulting from brain damage from a stroke. I would love to avoid the cold and have it easy, but I don't. I have a choice to make every day. Am I going to sit around here and complain? Or am I going to make shit happen and fight the challenges that pain throws at me? If you want a meaningful life, you will choose to fight pain for yourself and the people around you. Pain is temporary, but you're more than pain. You're more than your negative thoughts. You're powerful, unstoppable, and ready to begin the journey to become the best version of yourself. Because at the end of the day, pain ain't got nothing on you.

WAR WOUNDS

OUR SCARS ARE SYMBOLIC OF THE STRUGGLES WE HAVE SUR-
VIVED. Some scars look hideous, and we do everything we
can to hide them. Others look badass, and we want to show
them off.

I have scars from treatment. Each scar holds a lot more
content than people may think at first glance. The subtle
scar along the left side of my nose holds a horrific story
that shocks people when they ask, but people would never
assume that cancer was the answer to their question.

Let's say there's a large man walking across from you. He
has large purple and red scars running along his arms. As
you watch him walk, you notice people are actively avoiding
him. Their eyes see the scars and dart away.

Seconds later, a little girl runs up to the man and hugs
him, yelling, "Daddy! Daddy!" The people realize at that
moment that he isn't scary. He's a normal loving father. The
moment people see this, the tension lightens in the room. A
couple of people even crack a smile.

Our scars can not only create insecurities within ourselves but within others who see them.

If you have insecurities, it's important to own that scar. If that mark represents a traumatic event, it's your job to start loving yourself for being a warrior. You made it through hell, even if you were lucky, and you feel like you did nothing. It is your responsibility to recognize that it's a miracle that you did make it and that you have an opportunity to do good in the world. It's a battle scar. Keep on fighting like every day is your last.

Most importantly, don't jump to conclusions about who people are, based on their physical appearance. We sometimes base our first impressions of people on common stereotypes. We see a specific hairstyle or a particular clothing brand and label others with words like "jock" or "nerd."

Unfortunately, many label others before even getting to know them. And it makes me wonder, how many incredible people are we missing out on simply because we aren't willing to give them the chance to be themselves?

That nice man with the scars is worth your time. He brings happiness and smiles to the room, and what stopped you from getting to know him were the mental barriers that you built up to protect yourself from threats that don't even exist.

If you really want to see people for who they are and peel back layers, you're going to have to take a chance and ask the right questions.

Ask questions that are actually going to lead somewhere, like, "What have you been up to?" This question can lead to more answers lacking depth. The person could potentially respond, saying, "I've been working mostly."

Use this shallow answer as an entry point. You have now entered the doorway of a large mansion containing many experiences and memories. By entering, you have control over taking that conversation down a particular path.

Your response could be, "What do you do for work?"

Once you ask a question that could contain many possibilities, it's important to remember that your first impression of this person may not even come close to the occupation they answer with. For example, one of the guys that drove for Uber told me he had asked a client what she did for a living. He choked on his words when she responded, "I'm a stripper." That is one hell of an answer. I can't blame the man for being speechless. How do you even respond to that? "I'm a stripper too!"

"Omg! Seriously?!"

"Nope."

A couple of years after that Uber experience, I participated in a cancer support group. Once every two weeks, the group would get together and catch up. We ordered pizza and pop and had some laughs.

We all watched a video together where women showed their scars from their battle with cancer. Every scar was different and unique, and each survivor had her own story to tell. The common denominator was that all the women were proud of their scars, no matter how they appeared.

This made me realize that I needed to be prouder of mine.

I improved my confidence through self-talk and writing down positive reinforcements. I listed statements such as:

I am awesome
I am brave
I am smart
I am relentless
I am creative

I am hardworking.

I began recording this list every day. And eventually, I started believing what I was writing down. It became ingrained in me, a part of who I was and am.

Negative thoughts still come, but it was up to me to challenge those thoughts with the jurors in my head shouting what was "just." The jurors in our thoughts can become corrupt and can make us hate ourselves so quickly if we let them. It becomes easy to let them take control when we can compare ourselves to others on social media. And some may feel poorly about themselves when they feel like they don't live up to what others are posting online.

We are expected to work forty hours a week, raise a family, take care of ourselves, and to somehow, someway, learn to be happy. Damn, that is challenging.

Your job targets should be fulfilling. I know someone who's gone back to school to become a paramedic because he lost a loved one and wants to make a difference. He decided for himself what good he could provide for the world, and he chased it.

Nobody but you is going to push your life in a meaningful direction. But always remember that you don't have complete control over your thoughts and emotions. You will feel anger, sadness, and happiness. You are not immune to destructive emotions, and you're not weird for having negative thoughts either. We all feel them. It's an unfortunate part of life. But you must accept that having negative thoughts from time to time is a part of living. It's not our thoughts that define who we are. It's our actions.

Once you choose to take a meaningful direction, it's

also essential to be inspired by others. Also, take inspiration from yourself. You're an inspiration. You got this.

When you get inspired, something beautiful happens. A heart is grown full of passion and ruthless determination. You settle into what is true to you, and you essentially start to become what you were always meant to be, a winner. You will look back at the old you, smile, and think, wow, *look how far I've come.*

Life will continue to challenge you as you rise to take on the challenges it throws at you. Life will slash at your knees, break your courage, and make you feel uncertain. But the difference is, you will learn to adapt. Trust me. Stupidity comes across all of us. Regret leaks out from our pores. It can be hard to escape the negative, and it's time you acknowledge that.

War can bring out the worst in people, but it can also bring out the best and make heroes. So does life.

It is impossible to be happy all the time, and if you do know someone who is happy every minute of every day, I'm telling you they're either fucking delusional or bat shit crazy. It's critical to recognize that sadness will be a part of your life. Whether you want it there or not, it will forever be a shadow waiting to present itself.

There are medical plans, specialists who can offer their support and advice, and family and friends who will stand by you through thick and thin. There are also support groups that will relate to your concerns in a way that nobody else could ever understand. Those options are out there to help patch up the blows the world has dropped on you. They were there for me.

But for a while, there was something that really bothered me. The fact was that I had a visible tumour for months, but nobody caught it until it was almost too late. The sand in the hourglass was slowly but steadily draining, and I remained powerless. Each individual grain passed, and my time kept ticking. The nosebleeds continued, but "a nasal polyp" was the only answer given to me. Soon I began sleeping for hours, then days, then weeks. If it weren't for my parents, who carried me from place to place, I'd be dead.

Thank you, Mom. Thank you, Dad. Thank you for searching for answers even when they weren't within reach. When people at school thought I was faking being sick, you never gave up on me. And you still believe in me. No matter how hopeless or lost I felt, you stood by me. I wish more people were like you, but I guess that's what makes you both so special. You're incredible, and I would never have made it without you.

War wounds will cut all of us down, but always remember there are inspiring people out there. They just haven't realized how fucking badass they are, and neither have you.

BECOMING A WINNER

A SPECIAL PLACE. What's the first place that comes to mind? The house you grew up in? That pub you and your buddies always went to? The spot where you attempted to go camping but always miserably failed? Think of that place, the place where the magic happened. Let the memories flood you with the laughter, stupidity, or whatever you felt in that moment.

For me, I felt that magic biking in the desert or hiking to the tallest hill in Honolulu and watching the sunset. Experiencing those beautiful moments with the people you love is incredible. God damn, did I ever feel tired at the top, but it's the groans of pain my family made that come to mind, and boy, does it make me laugh.

But when I think back to those memories, magic comes to mind. The open desert dunes sprawled out in front of me. A playground of sand and rattlesnakes. That was my shit, and man, was it ever breathtaking. Those were the days. I took those moments for granted. But how was I supposed to know I was going to get cancer?

But a special place, where you venture to get a sense of "normalcy," where you feel at peace for being you.

In my months of recovery, I walked two miles to my favourite coffee shop. I appreciated the beautiful weather even more than I ever had before. Despite the exhaustion, I felt an extra skip in my step. I blasted music to and from. Crossing the familiar streets, I knew and loved.

My life had changed entirely, but the world hadn't. It was bizarre. It was brutal. How was I supposed to learn to live again? Regardless, every week, I walked to the shop and sat down with an iced chai latte; those were, and still are, my favourite. I guess you could call it my special place. It was my own personal safe haven. I was tired of being hurt, and I just wanted to feel safe and accepted. I found comfort in seeing the other kids my age studying and in sitting there with them.

For that hour, as I sat there, I felt like a regular 19-year-old guy again. I was no longer that kid who had cancer. I was a student and nothing more, nothing less. I still got looks of curiosity, but it was the closest to feeling normal I could get. I put on the headphones and read about history. I wasn't even that interested in it, if I'm quite honest with you. I just wanted to fit in. At that time, it's what I needed to do. I stuffed all the resentment I felt towards others deep down, and I left it there.

This special place, while comforting in the short term, was damaging in the long term. I returned to the coffee shop because it was relaxing, but there was more to it than just that. It allowed me to escape my current reality. I didn't have to live in a world where I was recovering from being sick because, in my head, I was better now. I was getting back to studying; I was getting back to being me. The issue was that the life I had was gone, and I wasn't willing to accept it.

After cancer and brain damage, nobody but my family and friends believed in me. Fuck, I didn't even believe in myself. I felt abandoned much of the time. The only way forward was to prove the non-believers wrong. Prove I was good enough. I'm not just here to play; I'm here to win. And while you may not be able to win with people, you sure as hell can win for you. What's truly remarkable is when you can utilize your own talents to help other people.

A great leader is a person who can bring ordinary people together to achieve extraordinary results. Helping other people is incredible. Bringing people together to make someone's day just a little bit better, we should all aspire to do that. Not for the gain of power but to better ourselves. Not to gain an unseen advantage but to put a smile on someone's face. Not to secure a win for yourself, but to secure a victory for us all. Meaningful teamwork can form bonds and friendships for life. It can also provide you with invaluable knowledge and insight.

When we lack the proper knowledge and insight, we can begin to pick ourselves apart, and it can become a constant mental battle. Believe me, I know. Nobody picked me apart and beat me up mentally more than me. It's easy to jump to shitty conclusions about yourself. It takes so much effort to build ourselves up and only a split second to tear ourselves down.

While I was sick, I watched a lot of global talent shows. Incredible acts from magicians to shadow dancers, there was always a spark of good entertainment.

One of the first things I noticed was the jealousy in

the comment section. Commenters were complaining about how it was unfair that these people were born with talents and how they, themselves, had been given nothing. However, some of these commenters don't realize that many acts on talent shows had to go through tons of judgment and rejection leading up to being on the show. Fans often only see the success. They never witness the external and internal struggles that come with it. Winners aren't born. Winners are made. It can be a long and hellish journey filled with many losses along the way.

The reason why there aren't more winners out there? People aren't willing to lose to win. It's all or nothing, and if "the all" isn't there. They settle for a boring life and spend the rest of it angry about how stupid it was that they never had their talents given to them on a platter.

Life doesn't work like that. Learn to love what you have, appreciate who you have. But never stop striving for improvement.

I kept seeing the group pictures that other people posted on social media when I was stuck in a hospital bed. It made me feel so alone and helpless. And there I was. Nowhere.

Then one day, I asked my parents if I could fill in the time with learning music. They were all in. I got a piano teacher, and I started learning how to play. I began with a basic C major scale. C to C with my left hand, and then again with my right. Due to the lack of feeling in my fingertips, it was hard and frustrating at times. My blind spot made it even harder. I couldn't see my right hand while playing most of the time. As frustrated as I was, I was not going to quit. I sure as hell felt like it at times, but there was a crucial reason why I never gave up. Music was always there for me, and I was always going to be there for it. It was as simple as that.

I had previous experience with guitar, and I worked hard. The result was good. Each day I made progress. It wasn't always fast, but it was progress nonetheless.

Learning to play music post-brain trauma was extremely difficult. How Stevie Wonder did it blindly, I will never know. As funny as that may sound, it gave me hope. If that man was capable of all that while blind, maybe I was capable of a lot more than I knew I was.

From that point on, my goal was to try my absolute best to prove to myself that I was capable of more than I knew.

I started learning Coldplay, Of Monsters and Men, and Linkin Park. I kept going up and down scales each day I could. And you know what? I loved it. It was an addiction and has become an integral part of who I am today. I would like to raise my glass to good music, folks. The memories it's given me.

I went to a rock concert after I found out I was cancer-free. Holy shit, I was never so grateful to be alive. I remember the rock screams echoing through the arena. All the lights that lit up the stadium. All the fans singing in unison, their eyes filled with love. And when we thought it was all over, they kept going. "You mother fuckers want more?!!" The singer screamed as the people in the crowd cheered in a chorus of applause.

They ended up playing an extra ten songs. They couldn't stop because they loved music so much, and that passion shone through.

The most successful bands are hard-working and

talented, but I don't think these are the key elements of a band's success. Those are important components that have made many bands winners, but it isn't "the" component. What it really is, is contagious passion.

Every minute of that concert was filled with excitement and a strong passion and love for music. These guys weren't in the music industry for fame or fortune. Nope, they're the real deal, and they're in it for the love, passion, and memories.

Many people are dissuaded from their true passions throughout life due to the ideals that society has laid out. Instead of asking for permission to be accepted, it's much more valuable to permit ourselves to be who we really are.

Our own society can prevent us from becoming what we were meant to be. There are countless potential business owners out there. But they threw it all away due to a lack of guidance, limited inspiration, or the drugs and alcohol they fell into.

The first step to becoming a winner is accepting that you have a lot of growing to do. This is a good thing, though! So, don't get yourself down.

Some develop a losing attitude, spending too much time feeling sorry for themselves, and it's gotten them nowhere. Find something positive to pour your time into, and then door after door will open. Don't chase glory and fortune. That will get you nowhere. What does your heart really want? Where do your talents line up with having the biggest impact? What does that impact look like? A laugh? A smile? Raising money for people in need?

Everything is getting more expensive as well. The price of many things are going up. For example, as seen on

Statistics Canada, gasoline at self-service stations were 95 cents per litre in January 2006. However, as of March 2021, the price is 125 cents per litre.[13] just ask your parents and your parent's parents. Many things used to be more afford-able—goodbye, sweet dreams, and hello, dear sweet debt.

Winning in a society that writes a prophecy for you to lose seems impossible. In my case, it was brutal. Life is already hard enough, add my neuropathy and blind spot to the equation: fewer people want to hire me because some employers may see me as a burden. It has made my life heartbreaking in so many ways. There were days when I looked at myself in the mirror after another failure, and I felt so frustrated. As frustrated as I got, my family always helped me get back in the game. Try and try again and again. And when trying wasn't enough, I still kept trying.

Then one day, I had an idea. I had a dream of inspiring somebody. to write a book sharing my struggles. Showing people that they are capable of more than they could ever possibly imagine. That everybody could quit on you, but if you didn't quit on yourself, there was always hope. I started writing and researching. It felt so right, so I kept coming back to it; some days, I stayed up till three in the morning coming up with ideas or reading about others' experiences through books and online articles. And for the first time in a very long time, I felt like myself. I felt like me. It not only felt right but necessary. How did I know it was right, you ask? It's simple. I felt like a winner.

---

13 Statistics Canada, *"Monthly average retail prices for food and other selected products,"* Last updated April 29, 2021, https://doi. org/10.25318/1810000201-eng.

THE BOY

A BOY SPENT DAYS LOOKING FOR OPENINGS IN THE LOWER WINDOWS OF A CASTLE. The inside of the castle was within view. He could almost taste it. Right there on the other side of the portcullis. The open main bailey awaiting him.

Beams of flashing sunlight slipped through the puffy white clouds, flooding the castle in a spectacle of a bright dancing orange glow. Perfect it was, and tall it stood. Its tallest towers reached like arms forty meters high, just scraping the closest edge of the sky.

Guards stood, both day and night—men armed with arrows scanning the country with lazy eyes. Day and night, they stood waiting, standing guard. Time went on, and nothing changed. The guards continued their rounds, royal guests flowed in and out of the castle walls, and the boy remained a poor boy begging for food in the streets of a town nearby.

The knights would joust every day in a flat field west of the castle walls. Their armour shone brightly even on the darkest of days. Angry storm clouds rolled in, flashing with spectacular bursts of current, shaking the ground with enormous booms. While many took shelter, the boy stood in the rain. Cold he was, hungry he was, but watch he must.

Knights fell, and knights rose. The boy could hear no sound of the battles fought vigorously below as the sky raged above him. Hooves pounded the ground. Mud flew high, and metal met metal. One man was unseated, his body flying through the stormy air. Time seemed to go slower at that moment, the boy thought. It was as if the king had a stopwatch that allowed him to do so. He was the king, after all.

King Henry was believed to have a pact with the gods. A brotherhood of sorts. At least that's what the boy's mother had told him.

The boy did not understand any of it. He had always wanted to be a knight ever since he could remember. Every opportunity he got, the boy would go and watch the knights joust and train, plan how he would sneak past the guards, and prove himself worthy of knighthood to the others. He pictured his mother there watching him, proud with a beaming smile and bright wide eyes. He only saw love in her eyes, only love. He had his mother's eyes—a deep ocean blue.

The rain continued to pound the ground around him. His mother would be worried sick. He had been sneaking out of the shack for a while now. He dreamed of becoming a knight, so much so that he disobeyed his mother's safety regulations on the regular. "You're all I have left, Ollie! Don't run off." She would tell him sternly with a finger pointing hard into his chest. She was always angry afterward, but that was because she cared. She cared about him on his good days, his bad days, and the ugly ones too. His mother had always been there for him. When Oliver had been on the street corner begging for money, and others had refused to even look at him, she was always there to welcome him home. Many days tears would line her eyes when she saw him. "Oh, Ollie, I'm so lucky to have you!"

In the village, there were other boys and girls like Ollie. His friends James and Amelia often trained together. There was an abandoned barn in the town they would walk to for training. It was about a mile downhill, but it was perfect. The three of them used small tree branches they had found on the outskirts of the village. The three friends each took turns fighting one another.

Amelia was quick and agile. She danced like a panther slipping in and out of the boy's reach—her dark brown hair tossing from left to right.

James was larger than Oliver. Stalky and strong, but awkward he was. Amelia would often toy with him in the barn. Walking circles around him. She took every chance she could get to take pokes at her opponents. It was tricky to parry her due to her speed and agility. But all you had to do was get one good hit at her leg, and she would slow down to a manageable pace. It still was not easy, though it became easier.

James, on the contrary, would not take pokes. He would swing with massive amounts of power and strength. While dodging his strikes was relatively easy, you never wanted to get hit by him.

The three of them never had long to practice as they had to return to the streets. In those moments of training, though, Oliver always felt so happy. He completely forgot about how poor he was or even how cold he felt. All he saw were his two best friends and the branches between them.

When Oliver returned to his mother, he would share his frustrations. How unfair it was that he could never be a knight. That there would never be a day where he could fight and smile proudly. That's when Oliver told his mom everything. About the barn, the training, and why he always snuck out. It all poured out of him like the pain that had poured down on him in the fields. But just like the rain, it all felt refreshing. It was needed.

The boy's body shook when he told his mother. She took hold of him and hugged him tightly. She pulled away and set her hand on Oliver's shoulder softly. She looked her son in the eyes, a tear streaming down from her blue eyes. "Tomorrow, I want you to go back out to the barn with James and Amelia."

"But why? I thought you hated when I snuck out?"

"Oliver, I discovered a long time ago that you can't change people. You can try, but people are who they are. And this is who you are. The next opportunity you get, I would love for you to go back out there." She smiled softly, glanced down momentarily, and whispered. "It's what your father would have wanted."

The following day Oliver ran out into the sunshine, beaming when he saw James and Amelia talking in the streets. Oliver made his way through the muck of the streets and navigated through the many villagers passing by. "Looking short there, Oliver!" James exclaimed. All Oliver could do was smile back at him.

As they began to walk, Oliver told them about how

he had opened up about everything to his mother. "You didn't!" gasped Amelia. "Oliver, you could have gotten into so much trouble! What were you thinking?!"

"I'm tired of hiding Amelia! It feels so stupid! I want to be me. It's what my father would have wanted." And with that, the three friends ran off towards the barn. And in that moment, three warriors ran across the fields shining as bright as the bravest knights.

BREAK FREE

As KIDS, MANY OF US HAVE OUR PARENTS READ US STORIES. From a very young age, we develop a habit of picturing things in our minds and eventually build our own self monologue inside our heads. This monologue, of course, varies from person to person.

Every child grows up with different circumstances and is unique in their own way. That's what makes them an individual. Because of our unique situations, every one of us has a different approach to self-talk. One child may develop a cocky voice and, as a result, act cocky.

We also formulate particular skills due to this voice, as well as the voices of others. Some become good with numbers and may eventually pursue a career in finance, while others find themselves amid creation, leading to the beginning of a new business idea. Unfortunately, we don't all end up pursuing what we really want.

I had someone in the gym start a conversation with me. It eventually led to the question, "What do you want to do with your life, man?" This question caught me off guard. Fuck, I was only twenty at the time. Regardless, I took a shot at the question. I told him that I was mainly focused on online classes and getting myself into better shape. I don't remember where the conversation went from there. I do, however, remember the walk back home. I was still shocked that someone would ask me that after five minutes of conversation. Damn. "What do you want to do with your life?" How on earth was I supposed to answer that question? I didn't even know what I was eating for dinner yet. It sure made me think, though. There was no way I would figure that out when I had more room to grow and many more things to learn.

The question itself was impossible to answer at the time, but here's what it did do. I started thinking about what activities were beneficial to me. I thought about the gym. My goal was to put on more weight. I wanted to pursue my goals instead of waiting around. Not only would that be beneficial to my state of mind, but it would also benefit my health and make me a stronger, happier, and healthier human being. And after cancer, there was zero doubt about that being a fantastic thing. It was not only wanted but needed. I felt fantastic after working out. The feeling of walking out on a warm day blasting music on the way to a workout. Damn, was it good.

I also thought about eating better. My brother had made lots of progress at the gym due to a good work ethic and a great diet. And I wanted to make some healthier choices after I saw what he was doing. So, one day I just decided. It was that simple. I didn't need an excuse like a new year's resolution to make the change. Nope, right here, right now.

Before this change, I wasn't eating horribly, but I certainly could have been eating better. Lots of pasta with cream sauces. Some burgers, the occasional pizza here and there. Keep in mind, I did still eat healthy meals, but I sure could have limited the processed foods. Processed foods are high in fat, sugar, and salt. We love it and with fast food delivery. It's an all-you-can-eat buffet. And let's be honest, we're not all eating healthy when we use these apps.

When I was hospitalized with cancer, the doctors were puzzled because I was a healthy young man in their books. Adding a bunch of unhealthy food that lacked the proper nutrients and vitamins will get you in the long run. It may even get you in the short run too. You are what you eat, and that goes for your mood too. Mood and food rhyme for a reason, and often after eating fast food, I don't feel so great.

After I eat fast food, I feel tired and unproductive. After changing what I ate, I saw results, and they were good.

My endurance increased, and I was able to get more done in one day. I also found long runs easier to achieve. It made sense. Food is what fuels our body, and I was better as a result. I regained my strength faster after those brutal rounds of chemo. I could deadlift more, squat more weight, and study for longer periods of time. Learning to cook instead of just buying a cheeseburger was definitely the right move.

As a kid, I never liked putting any effort into what I ate. Because it was so much easier to pour out a bowl of cereal and call it a meal, I changed that. And damn, do I ever feel better and more energetic. I went to work out, came home, and got my carbs with my oatmeal. Sure, it doesn't sound as exciting as buying pizza. But how I felt physically was more exciting to me.

Now on the flip side, we all like to have a good burger from time to time or binge on unhealthy food. And that's perfectly okay! It's just important to remember that too much of a good thing can be bad. Everything in moderation, people. Everything in moderation.

I also thought about this book I was writing. Most people who dream of writing a book quit halfway. Either from lack of motivation, fear of judgment, or fear of failure. When it comes to taking risks, it can be scary to put yourself out there. Although at times, I was nervous or didn't feel motivated. I kept going. Quitting halfway would have bugged me.

But why do we quit? Is it the worry of failure or looking like a moron that stops us? While that might be part of the reason. I don't think it's THE REASON. Why do we quit? Because we're afraid of facing who we really are.

We all judge people from time to time. Judging people is completely natural. The issue is the way that we're doing it. Our cell phones give us the power to judge anyone at any moment in time. Remember that voice in our heads I mentioned earlier? Every time our phone goes off, we get excited. *I wonder who texted me?* We feel happy when we get a text or likes on our social media accounts. From my own experience, I can say this is a real thing and a problem in our society. Especially with millennials.

When I posted pictures of my cancer journey to my social media account, it originally started as a way to share my story and to help others. But it quickly turned into an addiction. It was nice seeing all the likes and comments pop up, so I pursued it. The support from others definitely helped, but it gave me a sense of an identity, a fake persona. I was remembered by many of those people as the guy who had cancer.

Here's what sucks about that. I'm more than that. Many people didn't see past the online persona I had created. So, I stopped posting, and instead, I put my time into improving myself and hanging out with friends and family.

Once I distanced myself from social media, I noticed quite a few things. Social media is like a teleporter to a fantasy land. When you hate the real world, just hop in the teleporter, and fly into another. Welcome to the magical land of dopamine hits, superficial identities, fake angles, false information, and pictures of people on the vacation you wish you were on. Of course, not all of it is fake, not at all. But why spend so much time on social media when there is a real, amazing life waiting for you?!

People often post the perfect picture with the best angle, best smile. Well, you get it, best everything. It gives the impression that people are always happy. Nothing but smiles and laughs. Here's the thing, life is not like that at all. Not even close.

I celebrated my nineteenth birthday in the hospital with cancer. My mom made my birthday so much more bearable. She spent 500 dollars and bought me a Nintendo Switch to play games on. Thanks, mom. After all the puking and gagging. After all the stress that had built up inside of me. That made my day.

At that moment, I was dying to get back to school. I just wanted to be a normal kid again. I wanted to walk through a university with a new pair of shoes and a bag filled with books. That would have made me so happy. It was hard to see the people I knew posting videos of partying, school, and travelling. And there was no way to escape any of it. I was tied to my chemo pole, stuck in a room, at the end of the hallway, on the third floor.

Days were tough, but this wasn't how I imagined my nineteenth birthday. I should have been at the bar with my pals getting drunk and listening to great music. But here I was in a bed on the third floor at the end of the hall.

I thought about the things I could have been doing if I wasn't in the hospital. I imagined myself Snowboarding at Lake Louise with my family. Freezing our asses off and then sitting by the warmth of the fire after pigging out at a restaurant. Or walking around Phoenix shopping without a care in the world and going to another basketball game. Anywhere but here, here wasn't fun.

The point is, social media can be a great thing, but only if used in moderation. It becomes unhealthy when you need it to convince other people that you're beautiful, smart, or funny. This one personality trait, in turn, becomes your whole persona. And many people will define you as that one word. Essentially you become the online persona that you created.

And as mentioned before, Social media can be a gateway to comparing ourselves to other's online personas and feeling sad when we don't feel like we live up to everything happening around us.

No wonder so many of us are insecure when we have access to other's lives with a swipe of our phones. A day comparing ourselves to others, when we should be working on developing ourselves and improving our relationships with others.

Step one to security is accepting that you've got a problem. Denial won't help you. I've witnessed people who are in denial. It isn't pretty. Get up, look your phone in the face and move on from it. You got this. You have to believe to achieve. I'm here to tell you that your social media habits may be holding back your potential to grow and could be a significant cause of your insecurities.

When I was hooked on social media, many of my priorities were out of whack. Before I limited my time on it, I was doing all the wrong things. I wasted hours looking at memes, comparing myself to others, and feeling shitty when someone was in the Bahamas, and I wasn't. Shit, the list goes on, but I think you get the point. Stop trying to outlive the lives of others and start living the life you were always meant to live. Your life.

And with social media, you're not only selling yourself; you're selling yourself short. You are so much more than an online profile. You're incredible, but instead of spreading your wings, you've been tied down to an online profile that ties your self-worth with what others think about you. It's time to put down the phone and accept that you're fucking awesome, no matter what. Sure, you're not perfect; you've made mistakes, but here's the thing. Who hasn't?

The best piece of advice I can give you is to get involved in your life. Sports teams aren't for everyone (and they weren't for me). I loved kickboxing, but volleyball and soccer just weren't my thing. So, I kept working out and hitting bags. It just felt right. If you have doubts about what you're doing.

Sometimes a change is what you need.

It can be scary to mix things up. But who knows what extraordinary life you're missing out on? Don't look at me?! That awesome life is awaiting you, but it's your job to find it. Nobody else will do that for you but you. Your loved ones will help you along the way, but it is key that you recognize this. Your friends and family are there to support you but not to carry you to the finish line. The idea that there will be someone to save you is an idea you should not rely on. This isn't Brad's or Kevin's marathon. This is your life and your marathon. Own the run and own the fuck out of being you. That's an order.

We have become very reliant on our phones. Many have developed an impulse to reach for it when it buzzes. We don't even think. It just happens. It's hard to enjoy anything when everybody around you has their phone on their mind. It becomes increasingly harder to live in the moment when we crave for life on the web— Interconnected by a bombardment of information. There's too much stuff going on. People can't even filter it out anymore.

Our phones (in a way) have become a fifth limb on our body. We can't walk anywhere without it, We take it to the washroom, even though it's not even necessary. It's intertwined in our own identities, and in many cases, *is* our identity.

We all need breathing room. And it's perfectly fine to use our phones to text friends, family, and use social media. It's amazing that you can reach anyone you want in a matter of seconds. Anyone can bring people together for a good cause or stand up for what they believe in. Big or small, you can have a voice and a narrative. And with such a big world to explore with so many options, there are many people you can follow.

Perhaps an athlete who posts workouts that fans find helpful, which is amazing. It's incredible when someone is knowledgeable or talented at a skill and decides to spread that knowledge to help improve the lives of others. The fans who learn can then pass on that information to friends and family. The circle of giving just keeps on giving.

Other people spread positivity on social media. Now sadly, not all of this is genuine. You, of course, must take certain sites and profiles with a grain of salt. But there are some fantastic people spreading joy online and reaching thousands of people every day.

There's a waitress who has served my family and me a couple of times now. Most waiters are trying their best, and I gotta give it to them. It's a tough job. It's fast-paced, stressful, and they sometimes have to deal with some really shitty people. What blew my mind was how happy she looked, how big her smile was, and how she treated others around her. She was amazing. It made me think, *God, why can't more waiters be like her? Why can't more people be like her?*

Speaking of great people, let's talk about great T.V. characters. Ever watch a show that made you laugh so hard that you cried? A show where you were so invested in the characters that you felt like you knew them?

Throughout my journey, shows were a big part of my healing process. There was one show that I loved to watch every day. And even though it was just a T.V. series with actors, it somehow felt more real to me than any other show I had ever seen. Maybe it was because the actors were all getting along great, or the chemistry was just there. Whatever it was, I kept coming back to watch more. And now, cancer-free, I still go back. And it is these stories that helped me pass the time on my journey. They allowed me to break free from all the chaos, stress, and negativity in my life. And when freed from that negativity. My mind opened up to more possibilities.

I think that is something that would help us all in many areas of our lives. What if we were more open to working things out in our relationships? Maybe the rate of divorce would be lower? I could be completely wrong, but it's worth a thought. Maybe, what's holding us back is the lack of embracing other's ideas and becoming self-righteous with our own beliefs? Perhaps we need to be a bit more open about who we are? Maybe our relationships would be better as a result? And at only twenty-two years, I'm aware that I lack experience. It's just some food for thought.

When people in my life opened up to me about their own personal struggles, it only made our bond stronger. It's so important to have at least one person who knows you for you. A person that you can trust without hesitation or doubt. True trust is such a powerful thing. And when you got that group of people or person you trust, God damn, is it ever good. And oh boy, do you ever feel free.

NEVER QUIT

IT'S EASY TO QUIT. What makes it so easy is the accessibility. You can do it anywhere at any time. A flick of a switch, the pull of a chord, and it's all over. That's all it takes.

There's always a price to pay. A sacrifice of time and money in order to get things moving. A sacrifice in pride. Doing what you believe can often go against the common belief of others. Others may think you're delusional or even insane for chasing a goal with hunger and determination. And who knows, maybe you are a bit crazy? Quite often, creative or intuitive thinkers have a knack for thinking outside the box.

As people, we often overestimate the chance of losing and underestimate the chance of winning. The human mind gets wrapped up in possibilities of loss. It's easy to lose and hard to win. You don't have to try to lose. That's what makes it so easy. But what really hurts is second place. When you were so close to beating them all, but one person had the edge on you. It weighs heavily on the mind. Even though the medallist came home with silver, they still didn't achieve their goal of being "the best."

"The closer we are to winning, without actually winning,
the worse we feel."
— Christopher Sean Stewart

To feel better about losing, we try to rationalize. Make excuses, blame our circumstances, equipment, or coaches. We do this to protect our egos so that the loss doesn't hurt as much. And loss hurts.

Many don't live up to their potential because they never lived the life they should have truly lived. They gasp for breath because they were never meant to be a lawyer. You were meant to go into real estate. As a result, you're a good lawyer, but not a great one. While you could have been a superstar in the real estate market.

It's astonishing how many people end up on the wrong path. But of course, you must first find what's wrong in order to find what's right. We have to try on jeans to find the perfect fit and go on dates to find a suitable partner.

Others want us to quit not just because they're jealous but because they don't get it. They don't have the vision that we do. And how could they? There are discouraging people out there. Devoting yourself to a good cause or even an ideal can give you the structure you need to crush your goals.

I went back to my high school to volunteer at the bikeathon. The leadership program gave me a cause to align myself with. It gave me a sense of purpose and helped raise money and awareness for the many people struggling out there who never refused to quit.

There was always something special about that program and the people within it. I can't exactly quite describe it.

It was a feeling and a damn good one. My stresses and concerns would wash away in a split second. All the fear that I had. Gone. Volunteering at the bikeathon was what I needed. After all the pain I had gone through, I just wanted to be treated like a normal human being, and no matter how hard things got, I kept pushing on.

There's always a way forward. No matter what stands between you and your dreams, there's always a way. You may feel blinded, like you don't stand a chance in hell. But I never want you to quit. Never give yourself permission. It's unacceptable. We aren't our thoughts, and our thoughts go places. Voices in our heads tell us we are lost and are incapable of chasing our goals and dreams. It's up to you to counter that voice. Talk back to it, question it. Ask that voice in your head, "What gives you the right?" That voice in our heads is a nuisance, and it will always be there. That won't change. But you can change your approach to dealing with that voice.

Be vocal. Show that voice in your head who's in charge. "I can't do it!"

"Yes, I can." That's better.

> "Voices will always make sounds,
> but voices don't always need to be heard."
> — Christopher Sean Stewart

Put those headphones on and blast away. Blast away all the negative voices telling you that you aren't good enough. Prioritize your own voice inside your head and annihilate the negative ones that you come across. Do what you gotta do to make you believe in you. Self-belief is more powerful than you can imagine.

With the power of self-belief and a belief system, dictators are able to convince many people to do awful and atrocious things. They keep pushing their agenda at the cost of millions of innocent people's lives. They keep going and going, doing horrible things, but refuse to quit for all the wrong reasons. If one individual can convince a country that they must conquer and harm others, another's journey to develop positive self-belief should be a lot easier.

Just remember that it's a journey. You won't suddenly wake up feeling more motivated to make moves. That will happen gradually. There will be one or two days, occasionally, where you feel pumped up and ready to go. But it takes weeks or even months of practiced routine before you find something that works for you.

Having routines are an excellent backbone to have when a lack of motivation becomes apparent. I've got my alarm set now on many of my days. I wake up, eat oatmeal, make a chocolate peanut butter protein shake, and I get back to studying.

Having a routine not only makes your life more manageable, but you also get a rhythm going. And once you got that rhythm going, you'll attract people. In addition, having a routine will enable you to flow from one task to the next seamlessly. Of course, it will take practise, but it's possible.

I completely lost any semblance of routine when cancer became a part of my life. It keeps us busy. It distracts us from hardship and faults. Routine is satisfying as fuck once you've got it down pat. Wake up, study for a couple of hours, catch up with a pal, binge watch your favourite show, rinse and repeat. After two years of no routine, I can sure as hell tell you it's NEEDED. Routine keeps us grounded and centered. It provides emotional security so we don't get sucked down the wrong path.

When routine becomes lost, so do we. We feel a lack of purpose, unfulfilled, and useless. Trust me, I know. Despite my hard-fought battles and sacrifice, I felt useless at times. This feeling of uselessness spiraled out of control. I convinced myself I was useless and unwanted by others. Thus, the ideas in my head became my reality, and my reality turned into other's reality. How I saw myself (useless and broken) is how others saw me. A lot of it was my own fault. I believed something so deeply that I became the very belief I had created.

One day, we just have had enough. We can't take it anymore. We have to make a change in our lives. A lack of action is nothing. One step forward is everything.

It starts with a single step. I just woke up. It just happened. It was like waking up from a coma all over again. It was real. I had hated being me. I had hated being the guy who had gotten cancer. I was angry. I had my life taken away from me. It was unfair, and I never did anything to deserve a near-death sentence.

Coming so close to death was an odd experience. I don't remember seeing a light at the end of the tunnel or talking with anyone. It was just all black. I remember nothing. However, I will never forget the people who were there to fight with me right by my side. Even when all I saw was the darkness surrounding me when I was in a coma far from the life I had once had.

Man, it only seems like yesterday when I was surfing in Hawaii and watching a basketball game in Phoenix. Yesterday,

I was at peace. I was just a kid lost in the world, lost in the fun of it all. Yesterday looked so great. Did I end up here today because of destiny or fate? Today was brutal. Today was hard. But I keep marching on no matter the odds. I'll work every day that I can. I'll give every damn that I can. I'll march to the beat of my own drum and help others when they feel lost. Tomorrow is another day, a bright new beginning—a chance for change, an opportunity for winning.

Opportunity is there for the taking. But will you brave the risk that comes with it? Get on top of the podium, speak your mind, spread your wings, and fly?

Touch the clouds, do the impossible. Do whatever it takes because you will fail. You will hurt, but you will also win. There are locked doors waiting to be opened, rooms waiting to be discovered, knowledge to be gained for reasons other than fortune and fame.

Never let them get the best of you. Never quit on your vision; never quit on your ideas. And when your first idea doesn't work, move on to two, and then three. And when hesitation kicks in, jump in and believe.

Believe in yourself. Believe in a cause. Don't get distracted by fake news or what feels like a facade. Dedicate yourself to what you really love. Put in 10,000 hours, and then check your odds. Fail for laughter and fail for love. Take breaks when needed and ask for love when your heart needs feeding. Keep your eyes up and your chin down. Learn from your mistakes but learn to be proud.

Be proud of your strengths, but also your flaws. Learn to be real but act when necessary. You'll have days where you feel ordinary, but always remember you're extraordinary.

You're one in a million. So, don't quit on yourself if you have a vision. Have faith in your family, have faith in yourself, but never ever quit until you get your result.

We write music, judge ourselves, and quit. We feel self-conscious about our bodies and stop going to the gym. Instead of putting 10,000 hours into our craft, we make excuses when we could have learned to adapt. When we could be doing what we love, we give in to peer pressure when push comes to shove. I always like to think, "but what if?" What if we made a sacrifice today for tomorrow? Gained respect for ourselves and started treating ourselves the way we deserve to be treated. Give ourselves the benefit of the doubt when all we feel is doubt.

A part of us dies when we quit. Gone with the tide, it just ceases to exist. Where did that part of us go? Who knows? Probably in a better place, though. A place without the internal struggle, where it can be free, where it can become what it needs to be.

It's unfortunate that the greatest part of a person can become a lost souvenir in the wind. What could have been a strong, unique individual, instead, becomes something different.

I never asked for cancer. If it were up to me, I'd be studying, working, and partying. But I had a fight to win and a life to live. And through trial and error, I would succeed.

The bravest thing you can do is make a choice. A choice to change. Rewrite who you are and who you're going to become. Life is a never-ending battle. It's time. Time to show life, the never-ending battle you can bring. Go for that promotion. Fucking grind. Work your ass off. Fail to succeed, succeed till failure. The key to life isn't happiness. It's a routine filled with every possible outcome and emotion. Expect nothing and accept everything.

We all have the ability to get it done. To commit ourselves to what needs to be done. Turn on that inspirational video that makes you feel like you can bench press a bench press. That's right, get into that shit. Feel the waves of vibration—the waves of happiness, upsets, and struggles. Get knocked down by the ball time and time again. But always get up. Just like in a bowling alley, you'll feel like a pin. No arms, no legs. It's a struggle being a bowling pin. But that's why we have "the claw," my friends. The claw is your closest mates and family—the people who refuse to see you quit on yourself.

Most of us are not at an end or a beginning. We're somewhere lost in the middle. We're ordinary people trying to survive, barely getting by and paying our bills, completely unfulfilled. It's like we've been dropped in the middle of the Sahara without a fucking compass. No wonder we're lost! Have you ever been lost in the Sahara before? Nope, neither have I. Maybe one day Chris...maybe one day...

What inspires many of us are ordinary people who have done extraordinary things. It's incredible to see that it's possible to become something more. To rise above and make something of yourself.

I want you to realize that there's a strength in you. A power that you might not even know that you have. What is that power? It's courage. The courage to keeping going. The courage to keep fighting. The courage to not quit. Never quit, people. Lose, take breaks, make mistakes, but never, ever give up.

HOME

A PLACE TO REST YOUR HEAD, WHERE THE PRESSURE RELEASES, A PLACE WHERE YOUR FEAR AND WORRY EASES. Where your vinyl's play in times of needing. The place of rest and the studying of tests. Life is a test in itself, filled with joy, truth, and lies. It all gets so hard, but if we just close our eyes. Forget about our worries of the past, present, and future and come to peace with ourselves. Take our shots, earn our pride, build a home for ourselves in the prairie for our family to find. A home, however, is more than a physical place. It's a sense of belonging that one can't erase. We've become fixated and want more until more isn't enough, and we become stuck without cause, purpose, or form. You'll search far and wide for answers that don't exist. You'll make excuses when you could have learned to commit.

But when it all comes down to it, it starts with you. Take care of yourself, find a hobby. Strive for a job that gives you a sense of belonging. Take the time that you need and treat yourself right. As short as life is, so much more can be done that is right. Right for you, right for the people you love, right for the people struggling down below and up above.

Many more are depressed, but why? Is it due to social

media and time lost before our eyes? Is it something less? Or something more? I hope for a better tomorrow. A tomorrow where we aren't afraid to be who we really are. Where criticism is constructive for the means of better lives and health. But in order to learn, a bird must leave the nest. It must tempt fate in times of struggle and regret. A bird must fly, but a bird must fall. For what goes up, must come down.

We bet on stocks and companies from left to right. We take a left when we should have taken a right turn. Lost we get. We pull out a map or a compass to get a sense of direction, a place to rest our heads.

Just take me home; take me home, away from the hospital and all the flashing lights. Take me back to when school and friends were my worries and when it all felt so simple and boring. Did this just all happen? Or is there a reason for our stories? Is there a purpose for you? Is there one for me? I believe there is, but it will be hard to find. You'll look high and low, far and wide. Lessons will be learned, and the dots will align.

From one day to the next, some will win, some will fail, but it's only through failure that we'll learn to prevail. Struggles will come and rise from the ashes. But only through facing your fears will the terrifying vision come passing.

There's a dream to be sought after. It won't be ideal, and it won't be picture perfect. It won't be something you ever could have imagined. A dream doesn't have to stay a dream, and it can become more than a vision. So, hold your head up high and keep believing in your decisions.

Take pride in a clean and organized house that leads to a clear state of mind. And when presented with a challenge, put up a good fight. There are 10,000 reasons to quit, 10,000 reasons to keep trying, but never give up because it's worth fighting.

Cancer crushed my body and mind, but not my spirit. I'm not the smartest, and I'm not the quickest. I compared myself to others when I felt I had nothing. No job, no school, and no sense of belonging. But when I fell, my family picked me up, and so I continued to fight.

I went to schools and told kids it was possible, and I'm telling you the same. You can do it. I believe in you. I think you are an incredible person. There are seven billion people, but only one of you. You are filled with so many undiscovered talents, but first, you must learn to love what you have.

Love your family and friends for their perfections and flaws. Learn to love yourself even when alone and lost. Continue to learn and continue to grow. When I felt lost, I came back home. To rediscover myself and rewrite who I was. And with enough time, I found my purpose and cause.

It was my mother and father who believed in me when I couldn't see a way out, my friends who gave me a laugh when I felt doubt, my grandparents who drove me from scan to scan, brothers who made me laugh and told me that I can. And when I felt lost, with no sense of where to go. I picked up my bags, and I came back home.

LIFE GOES ON

A CANCER SURVIVOR NAMED KEVIN HAD TOLD MY DAD AND I THAT THE MOST CHALLENGING PART OF CANCER WASN'T THE BATTLE ITSELF BUT THE READJUSTING AND REINTEGRATION BACK INTO A NORMAL LIFE.

For me, staying focused was one of the hardest parts. It becomes easy to let the emotions from a cancer experience overwhelm you. I would get fixated on a troubling thought or memory, and all parts of me would stop. What I needed to be reminded of were the obstacles I had overcome.

Over the past year and a half, significant progress has been made through brain and physical therapy, progress that I was damn proud of. What made these therapies so convenient was that they gave me something to do. A distraction to help keep my eyes up and head forward.

Like I mentioned earlier, cancer made me feel unordinary when all I wanted to feel was ordinary. My past kept me from moving on. Part of it was I still had to deal with a lot of the things I mentioned earlier. Like the feeling of fear, chaos, and pain that came with it. Or the feeling of being left out of a life I felt like I should have been living.

Over those months, I took time each day writing out the

thoughts I had. I stored those thoughts away and accidentally came across what I had written months later. A lot had changed, and it made me realize how far I had come.

Before, I had felt like I had been cheated in many ways for the prior life I had lost. I felt jealous when I saw others living the life I wished I was living. It was vital for me not to deny those emotions but to deal with them slowly but surely, by writing them out, challenging them, and asking questions.

It was quite tricky. Soldiers come home haunted from things they've seen, and I, in my own way, had to get over what I saw and felt in the hospital.

When I was on my third round of chemo, I decided to go for another one of my walks along the third floor at the Cross Cancer. Along the hall, I slowly walked with Paul the chemo pole towards the small kitchen cupboard. It was very tiny. There was only enough room for a fridge, a sink, and some cupboards along the wall.

Two people could be in there at once, but it was still a bit of a squeeze. I had gone in to check for snacks. Sometimes you could find some pretty good food, like a pizza. It was rare but still possible to find.

I walked in, eager to get my eyes on the inside of the fridge. When I walked in, another man was standing in the room. He said hello, and we started talking. The first thing I noticed was how healthy he looked. There was no sign of fatigue or pale skin, so surely, he must be visiting a loved one. I, on the other hand, was weak, skinny, and whiter than a ghost. So, he knew where I was at.

Let's call him Gord. Gord was one of the nicest guys I've had the pleasure of meeting. Everything about this man made me feel better. Within seconds I knew that I liked him.

Gord then asked me how I had ended up here and what type of cancer I had. I filled him in, telling him about the nosebleeds, the emergency brain surgery, the surgeries that followed, along with the five rounds of chemo and twenty-seven days of radiation. I had gotten fairly used to answering this question. It had sort of become mindless and routine. Gord was shocked by what I had told him. He offered me his hand and shook mine with a firm grip.

When talking to others in hospitals, I often ask the same question, "why are you here?" The answer can often be heartbreaking, like a loved one expected to pass in a couple day's time. And in those crushing moments, I do the only thing I can think of. I reach in and give that loving person a hug. I can see it in their eyes. I can see how much these people love their friends and family fighting for their lives. I wish there was some magical word I could use to make their pain go away. Because I wanted nothing more in those moments than to free people of the physical trauma so that they could continue living the life they should have been living. But sadly, not everyone makes it.

It's hard when we have to move on from something we love or someone we lost. It feels so unfair when something terrible happens, but you're never given the reason why. I know many people who believe in a God, lots who don't, and many somewhere in between. It doesn't matter where somebody lies along that spectrum. As long as their belief system isn't harming anyone else, there's no reason why a Christian shouldn't be able to hang out with an atheist. By having a closed mind, we are only limiting our knowledge and our sense of self. Life will go on no matter what you believe in. The Earth will continue to spin, and the sun will continue to rise.

I didn't pray while going through treatment, which may surprise many of you. Most of the patients I talked to prayed religiously. It wasn't that I didn't believe in a God because I am surely open to the possibility. I needed not to have faith in religion to beat cancer but instead believe in myself and the fight I would bring. That is how I won my battle. Through love, support, and self-belief.

When I began to question my self-belief, my family's love and support reaffirmed it.

The battle was brutal, but the recovery felt like a war. At the moment of writing this, I have cosmetic surgery in four weeks to replace the bone the cancer ate away. I'm pumped to finally get my nose fixed and move on with my life after not working or attending school for two years due to cancer. I know it will be challenging getting back into those things. But I will get back into work and come out of university with a degree.

It will be hard, but I'm ready to fight tooth and nail. The challenges won't stop, but nor will I. Life goes on, and so will I.

I used excuses like my nose, but it only held me back. I told myself I'd get back to making new friends and dating once my nose was fixed. Life went on, and I stayed sitting there as opportunities and windows passed by. I was completely ready for success, but I let my feelings get the best of me. Don't let the small finicky details hold you back. You're ready to do amazing things.

My journey was and still is difficult, much of the time. I have continued medical checkups every three months. I look forward to the cosmetic surgery I'm receiving to make life a bit easier to bear. But I will always continue to believe in myself, regardless of the situation. And I think you should give yourself permission to believe in you. Don't wait to appreciate, don't wait for the moment. Learn to love the moment for what it is and the people for who they are.

It's time to breakthrough your own thoughts. It's time for a new day, a new beginning, a new dawn. It's time to be who you were always destined to be. It's time to be you. It's time to breakthrough.

ABOUT THE AUTHOR

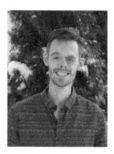

As a stage-four cancer survivor who underwent multiple rounds of surgery, chemo, and radiation, Christopher Sean Stewart had to learn to survive and to fight for his life and his future. Even though all the odds were stacked against him, with the help of his family and medical team, he has lived to tell the tale in this, his first book.

Christopher lives in Edmonton with his family.

BIBLIOGRAPHY

Bianconi, Eva, Allison Piovesan, Federica Facchin, Alina
    Beraudi, Raffaella Casadei, Flavia Frabetti, Lorenza
    Vitale, Maria Chiara Pelleri, Simone Tassani, Francesco
    Piva, Soledad Perez-Amodio, Pierluigi Strippoli, and
    Silvia Canaider. "An Estimation of the Number of Cells
    in the Human Body." *Annals of Human Biology* 40, no.
    6 (November 2013): 463-71, https://doi.org/10.3109/0
    3014460.2013.807878.

National Cancer Institute. "Cisplatin." Cancer Treatment:
    A to Z List of Cancer Drugs. Last modified October 7,
    2020. https://www.cancer.gov/about-cancer/treatment/
    drugs/cisplatin.

————. "Etoposide." Cancer Treatment: A to Z
    List of Cancer Drugs. Last updated July 19, 2019.
    https://www.cancer.gov/about-cancer/treatment/drugs/
    etoposide.

————. "Nerve Problems (Peripheral Neuropathy)
    and Cancer Treatment." Side Effects of Cancer
    Treatment. Reviewed January 15, 2020. https://www.

cancer.gov/ about-cancer/treatment/side-effects/
nerve-problems.

Parkin, Simon. "Has Dopamine Got Us Hooked on
Tech?." The Guardian, March 4, 2018. https://www.
theguardian.com/technology/2018/mar/04/has-dopa-
mine-got-us-hooked-on-t ech-facebook-apps-addiction.

Statistics Canada. "Monthly Average Retail Prices for Food
and Other Selected Products." Last updated April 29,
2021. https://doi.org/10.25318/1810000201-eng.